Colette Ray
Michael Baum

Psychological Aspects of
Early Breast Cancer

Springer-Verlag
New York Berlin Heidelberg Tokyo

KU-611-045

Colette Ray
Department of Psychology
Brunel University
Uxbridge
Middlesex UB8 3PH
England

Michael Baum
Department of Surgery
King's College Hospital Medical School
Rayne Institute
London SE5 6NU
England

Advisor
J. Richard Eiser
Department of Psychology
University of Exeter
Exeter EX4 4QG
England

Library of Congress Cataloging in Publication Data
Ray, Colette.
  Psychological aspects of early breast cancer.
  (Contributions to psychology and medicine)
  Bibliography: p.
  Includes index.
  1. Breast—Cancer—Psychological aspects.   2. Stress
(Psychology)   3. Psychotherapy.   I. Baum, Michael.
II. Title.   III. Series.   [DNLM: 1. Breast Neoplasms—
psychology. WP 870 R263p]
  RC280.B8R39   1985   616.99′449′0019   84-26849

©1985 by Springer-Verlag New York, Inc.
All rights reserved. No part of this book may be translated or reproduced in
any form without written permission from Springer-Verlag, 175 Fifth Avenue,
New York, New York 10010, U.S.A.

The use of general descriptive names, trade names, trademarks, etc., in this
publication, even if the former are not especially identified, is not to be taken
as a sign that such names, as understood by the Trade Marks and
Merchandise Marks Act, may accordingly be used freely by anyone.

While the advice and information in this book are believed to be true and accurate
at the date of going to press, neither the authors nor the editors nor the publisher
can accept any legal responsibility for any errors or omissions that may be made.
The publisher makes no warranty, express or implied, with respect to the
material contained herein.

Typeset by Publishers Service, Bozeman, Montana.
Printed and bound by R.R. Donnelley & Sons, Harrisonburg, Virginia.
Printed in the United States of America.

9 8 7 6 5 4 3 2 1

ISBN 0-387-96122-4   Springer-Verlag   New York Berlin Heidelberg Tokyo
ISBN 3-540-96122-4   Springer-Verlag   Berlin Heidelberg New York Tokyo

Preface

Physical illness cannot be effectively treated other than in the context of the psychological factors with which it is associated. The body may have the disease, but it is the patient who is ill. Research psychologists from a number of different backgrounds have, in the past few decades, turned increasingly to the study of physical illness, and there is now an extensive literature on preventive behaviors, the role of stress in the etiology of illness, the patient's reactions to illness and its treatment, and the physician-patient relationship. At the same time practicing clinical psychologists have extended their concern beyond the treatment of specifically psychiatric disorders, to include also the psychological care of people experiencing distress through illness or injury. Traditionally, these patients have tended to fall through the net, unless their distress is so great that it assumes the proportion of a psychiatric disorder that can then be treated in its own right. Because the physical disorder is the primary one, its existence has detracted from the salience of the very real emotional disturbance to which it can give rise. Moreover, emotional reactions in this setting, being the norm, seems to have been regarded as not meriting special attention and care. This situation is changing, and it is not just psychologists or psychiatrists who are responsible for the shift in attitudes. Within general medicine itself, there is now a renewed emphasis on the care of the whole patient and not just the disease. Nurses and physicians are themselves initiating research into psychological aspects of illness and its treatment, and they are increasingly taking these factors into account when deciding on treatment and the management of their relationship with the patient.

Cancer is an illness whose psychological implications have been more widely discussed than most, and breast cancer has been given more attention, at least from a research point of view, than other cancers. While this is the focus of this book, many of the topics dealt with have a more general application. All serious illnesses have some shared psychological implications, as well as specific ones dependent on the nature of the illness. Thus, we have cited research concerned not only with breast cancer directly, but also research dealing with cancer in general and with illnesses other than cancer.

We hope that this book will be of interest to surgeons, physicians, nurses, psychologists, psychiatrists, and other professions who care and provide support for the cancer patient. There are difficulties in writing for such a wide audience. The fields of both medicine and psychology have their technicalities, but where we have been unable to avoid jargon we have tried at least to explain the concepts and terms used. Finally, this is not a handbook, with explicit recommendations for patient care. Many of the issues addressed are complex and controversial, and each patient is an individual with her own specific needs and concerns and should be approached as such. What we have done is to present an outline of research and thinking, providing a framework within which the practitioner can make informed choices about the strategies to be adopted.

Where appropriate, we have used quotations from patients and from surgeons to illustrate the points made. These are mostly taken from interviews carried out as part of a project funded by the Cancer Research Campaign, on perceptions of breast cancer and its treatment and of the surgeon-patient relationship. They help to remind us that the dilemmas discussed in the literature are not abstractions, but are lived by the patient and by the clinicians who take on the burden of her care. The underlying issues are those central to the human condition, and brought to a focus in this situation: life versus death, autonomy versus compliance, striving versus passivity, and freedom versus fate. It is easy to focus on the failures, on patients' difficulties in coping, and on the inadequacies of the care that they receive. What is more remarkable is the fortitude and dignity with which many physicians and patients alike face the struggle and the challenges and disappointments that it presents.

Colette Ray
Michael Baum

Contents

1

Breast Cancer and Its Treatment

Over 12,000 women die of breast cancer every year in the United Kingdom. In the United States the figure is 34,000. It ranks as the commonest cancer in women and the commonest cause of death among women in the 35 to 55 age group. An individual woman in her lifetime stands a one in 14 chance of developing the disease, and there is even some evidence that the annual incidence and mortality are increasing slowly throughout the Western Hemisphere. Because of these disturbing facts and the very nature of the disease, the subject has become highly charged and emotional, so much so as to cloud rational discussion.

History

A lay person could be excused for believing that breast cancer is a new disease, when in fact it is probably as ancient as womankind. Cancer of the breast has been recognized as a disease process since the time of the ancient Egyptians, and an early papyrus described how it was differentiated from infectious mastitis. In those days no treatment was indicated other than cautery for the ulcerated tumor. Surgery for breast cancer was practiced by the ancient Greeks, but Hippocrates considered no treatment at all was superior to surgery, probably a very sensible opinion in those days. In ancient Rome at the time of Celsus, a primitive form of mastectomy was probably being carried out. In some ways Celsus also distinguished between early and advanced disease, and recognized the futility of surgery in the latter case. We can shudder to think of the suffering of these women in the days before anaesthesia and antisepsis, and the so-called Dark Ages must have produced a welcome respite from the surgeon's amputation knife. According to the doctrines of Galen who dominated medical thinking between the classical period and the Renaissance, black bile (melancholia) was the causal factor in the development of breast cancer, and special diets designed to avoid the accumulation of black bile were recommended. In addition, exorcism plus a variety of local applications were commonplace. It is perhaps salutory to remember that during the Third Century AD mastectomy was carried out not as a therapy but as a *punishment*, and poor St. Agatha was sent to her untimely grave after a bilateral amputation of her breasts.

Following the Renaissance, Versalius and Fabricus again recommended mastectomy with wide surgical excision of the tumor for breast cancer. Le Dran (1685–1770) recognized that the disease spread to the axillary lymph glands and advocated that these should be removed if enlarged. He was probably the first to describe the poor outlook associated with involvement of the nodes, and went on to advocate removal of the primary growth and the axillary nodes in continuity. It is difficult to judge the success rate of these procedures, since statistics of recurrence and survival were not formally collected. However, there is anecdotal evidence that some women survived these operations performed under such primitive circumstances, and went on to enjoy a normal expectation of life.

In the middle of the last century surgeons started to keep reasonable records of their experience in treating breast cancer, and Sir James Paget's experience (1853) of 74 cases treated by mastectomy, with a 100 percent recurrence rate within eight years, is probably typical of that era. James Syme (1842), writing in his textbook, *Principles of Surgery*, stated "It appears that the results of operation for carcinoma when the glands are affected is almost always unsatisfactory however perfectly they may have seemed to have been taken away. The reason for this probably is that the glands do not participate in the disease unless the system is strongly disposed to it and consequently their removal, however freely and effectively executed, cannot prevent the patient's relapse." These are highly significant comments. First, they indicate that some form of radical operations were being performed in an attempt to clear completely the affected glands, and, second, they illustrate that significant involvement of the axillary nodes was seen as indicative or symptomatic of a systemic disease. It has taken well over 100 years to recognize the wisdom of James Syme. In spite of his observations, surgeons persisted in their attempts to clear the axilla perfectly. It would appear that, before Halsted's description of a radical mastectomy in 1890, surgeons were already carrying out routine removal of the axillary nodes in addition to removing the breast. If we refer to Halsted's early publications concerning the results of radical mastectomy, we read of a high proportion of three-year "cures." His criteria for a cure would not be acceptable by today's standards. To get a true perspective of the long-term outcome of his methods of treatment, it is necessary to consult the records from John Hopkins Hospital in Baltimore between 1889 and 1931. During that period, 900 patients were operated on by Halsted or his followers. 6 percent died soon after surgery and the local recurrence rate was 30 percent. The 10-year survival rate was a very disappointing 12 percent so, although it could be argued that the introduction of the classic radical procedure improved local control, there is very little evidence that its introduction influenced long-term survival.

Between the early 1930s and the 1950s, there were apparent improvements in the results of treatment of breast cancer. There is little doubt that this was artifactual and resulted from better selection of patients submitted to mastectomy. For example, in the early 1940s, the Manchester staging system was described in England, with stage I and stage II representing the operable group of cases, stage III the locally advanced disease where surgery was doomed to failure, and stage IV the patient with obvious distant metastases. In 1943 Haagensen in America described the Columbia clinical classification, with stages A and B representing the operable group, and stage C the locally advanced disease. As a result of better and better selection, the 10-year survival rate following mastectomy improved from about 10 percent in the 1920s to about 50 percent in the 1950s. This figure of 50 percent 10-year survival following mastectomy has remained stubbornly fixed until the time of writing, in spite of all the apparent benefits of early diagnosis, improved surgical techniques and the use of postoperative radiotherapy.

Etiology

A woman with a first-degree relative who has suffered from the disease stands about twice the chance of developing breast cancer compared with the rest of the age-matched population, but factors other than heredity are also important. If the causes of breast cancer were fully understood, then it might be conceivable to prevent the disease by changing life styles and practices that foster the disease, or by identifying those women most at risk and treating them preventively.

It has long been recognized that there are striking differences in the incidence of breast cancer in different geographical areas, and in addition, there is also evidence that the natural history of the disease is different within these areas. Until recently, the most marked difference in incidence of breast cancer has been between the high rate in western Europe and the United States, and the extremely low rate in Southeast Asia. Curiously, the incidence of the disease among Japanese women living in Hawaii appears to be mid-way between that in Japan and that of the Japanese community living in the United States. From these and similar data, the general impression is that the more developed the countries are, in the Western sense of the word, the higher the risk. Thus, it appears that environmental factors act powerfully in determining which women are more likely to develop the disease, and, of the various environmental factors that have been considered, diet, a high-fat intake in particular, has been implicated.

Initial reports suggested lactation as another factor that would protect against carcinoma of the breast. More recently it has been demonstrated that it is child-bearing rather than lactation which plays the protective role. Nulliparous women over the age of 30 are the group most at risk, whereas women who have borne their children under the age of 25, whether they were subsequently breast fed or bottle fed, share the same degree of protection. It has also been suggested that the number of menstrual cycles occurring before the first pregnancy may be the ultimate determinant, and this might explain the difference in incidence of the disease between the developed and the developing countries. Thus, at one extreme, the young English girl on a more than adequate diet will start menstruating at the age of 11 or 12 and will perhaps postpone pregnancy until after the age of 25, whereas an undernourished Asian girl may not start menstruating until the age of 17 or 18 and will perhaps become pregnant at her second ovulation. Recently, there has been publicity regarding the apparent increased risk of developing breast cancer among young women under the age of 30 following prolonged exposure to the contraceptive pill before their first pregnancy (Pike, Henderson, Krailo, Duke, & Roy, 1983). This subject is still being fiercely debated as judged by the correspondence columns in *The Lancet* following its publication. At this time it would be prudent to issue a verdict of "not proven" pending the maturation of a number of current prospective studies of appropriate design. In the meantime, it is important to maintain a sense of proportion and to remember that the risks of unwanted pregnancies in young girls may well exceed the putative increased risk (for women under 30 years of age) of inducing breast cancer as a result of adequate contraception by the pill.

Pathology

Breast cancer arises from the epithelial cells lining the lactiferous ducts or constituting the lobule of the glandular portion of the milk producing apparatus. Pathologists generally recognize a preinvasive variety of each type of cancer, in which the malignant cells are confined entirely within the ducts or lobules in which they originated with no evidence of invasion into the surrounding tissues. These are described as intraduct cancer, or lobular carcinoma in situ. Untreated, there is good evidence that a high proportion of such cases will progress to frankly invasive cancer, but if excised at this stage in the evolution of the disease there is almost 100 percent cure. Lobular invasive cancers are relatively uncommon, perhaps accounting for 8 percent of all types, but are frequently associated with multiple foci of malignancy in the same breast or, for that matter, the opposite breast. Of the breast cancers seen in clinical practice, 90 percent are of the invasive adenocarcinoma variety arising from the epithelium of the lactiferous ducts.

The earliest detectable change produced by an invasive duct cancer is of a hard, ill-defined lump within the breast. As the cancer invades locally, it infiltrates the fibrous ligaments that support the breast tissue on the chest wall, pulling in the overlying skin to produce the characteristic and sinister dimple. It may also invade along the lactiferous ducts causing these to shrink and invert the nipple. Further infiltration will ultimately lead to fixation or ulceration of the tumor through the skin, while deep invasion fixes the cancer to the underlying muscles over the chest wall. Widespread infiltration within the breast may produce edema of the overlying skin, causing it to thicken and producing the appearance of orange skin (*peau d'orange*). Spread of the cancer into the axillary lymph nodes leads to the appearance of hard lumps in the armpit, and occasionally these deposits themselves can infiltrate and ulcerate the skin. These gross clinical changes have been used as a crude method of assessing outlook, and are referred to as the clinical stages of the disease. The earliest stages with the best prognosis are represented by a small palpable lump within the breast and no clinical involvement of the axillary lymph nodes. At the other extreme, locally advanced cancer fixed to the skin or the deep tissues with gross involvement of the axillary lymph nodes carries a gloomy prognosis.

The appearance of the cancer in the specimen of tissue removed at mastectomy is very characteristic. In the majority of cases, the tumor has a granular or gritty cut surface, with radiating spicules often giving the crablike appearance from which it earns its name. The microscopic appearance of breast cancer is also characteristic. The cancer cells appear in irregular columns or pockets of atypical cells scattered throughout a background of fibrous tissue. Cancer cells can demonstrate a whole spectrum of differentiation. At one extreme they may form recognizable ducts and tubules that retain sufficient characteristics of the structure of origin as to secrete mucus. These well-differentiated cancers carry an excellent prognosis. At the other extreme the cells are so undifferentiated that their origin is no longer recognizable. These cancers are described as anaplastic, or poorly differentiated, and carry the worst prognosis. The degree of differentiation of the cancer as judged by the pathologist is referred to as the grade of malignancy, and this, combined with clinical stage, can give a reasonable estimate of outlook. In spite of knowing the stage and grade of malignancy, however, breast cancer can still behave in an unpredictable manner, with extreme clinical variability, and this adds to the difficulty of assessing the impact of therapy. Some of the most exciting new developments in the subject concern the development of biological and functional profiles of individual cancers that may allow us more accurately to predict their behavior and thus to select therapy on a more rational basis.

Following local invasion by direct infiltration, breast cancer may express its lethal potential by invasion into the bloodstream through the venous system, either directly or indirectly through lymphatic venous communications. The commonest sites for early secondary involvement are the regional lymph nodes in the axilla or the mediastinum, but extensive lymph node invasion usually indicates that the disease has also spread widely within the circulation. Viable cancer cells disseminated in this manner may lodge in the skeleton, the liver, the lungs, or the brain, thus contributing to the patient's death in a number of ways (e.g., bone marrow failure, liver failure, respiratory failure). On many occasions, the first a woman knows about her breast cancer is when she presents to the doctor with such diverse symptoms as jaundice or spontaneous fractures of the long bones, with the primary breast cancer having escaped self-detection until the disease was already widespread.

Treatment

Until about 20 years ago the objectives of surgery for primary cancer were easy to define. It was hoped that with clearance of the last cancer cell from the breast and the regional lymph nodes the patient would be cured, and to this end the classic Halsted radical mastectomy, which removed the breast, the underlying pectoral muscles and the axillary lymph nodes, was the conventional treatment. Over the last 10 to 20 years, several clinical trials have compared radical forms of treatment with conservative approaches. In general, no one form of treatment has been demonstrated to be superior to any other as far as survival is concerned, but all trials have consistently demonstrated the poor outlook associated with the involvement of the axillary lymph nodes.

To summarize the current view, therefore, it is believed that, first, except in rare instances, the involved axillary nodes are not a nidus for tertiary spread of the disease, but merely symptomatic that the disease is already systemic. Second, the outcome of treatment is not determined by the extent of the original operation, but by the extent of the undetected metastases in the vital organs present at the time of diagnosis. For these reasons there has been a change in emphasis concerning the role of surgery, and this may be described as follows:

1. In selected cases where the disease is confined to the breast, surgery alone might be sufficient to achieve a cure.
2. In other cases where the disease has already spread, surgery still has an important role in achieving local control of the disease so that, even if the woman dies of metastic breast cancer, at least she is not distressed by a painful, infected, and ulcerated lesion on the chest wall.
3. Determining the pathological stage of involvement of the axilla is now considered to play an important role in the first surgical approach to the disease, in order more accurately to determine the prognosis for the individual woman. The importance of this step becomes clear when considering the role of adjuvant systemic therapy (see below).
4. It is likely to become increasingly important to have as large a sample of tumor as possible for more detailed histological and biological assessment. For example, modern techniques can measure the hormone responsiveness or dependence of the breast cancer, and this allows a rational exploitation of endocrine therapy.

Bearing these objectives in mind, a number of strategies are currently favored by most surgeons in the United Kingdom. First, the classic Halsted mastectomy has been more or less abandoned in favor of the modified (Patey) radical mastectomy. This spares the pectoralis major muscle while at the same time allowing full clearance of the axillary nodes. Some surgeons favor a simple (total) mastectomy, merely sampling the lymph nodes in the lower third of the axilla and then referring the patient for radiotherapy in those cases judged to have a high risk of local recurrence (i.e., those with large primary tumors, poorly differentiated cancers, or with positive axillary lymph nodes). Finally, in selected cases with small primary tumors, many surgeons are now adopting a policy of local excision of the tumor (commonly known as "lumpectomy"), sampling the lower axillary nodes, and then giving radical radiotherapy to the residual breast and lymphatic fields.

It should be recognized that a number of surgeons have for a long time been aware of the psychological sequelae of mastectomy and have leant toward conservative surgery with this in mind. As far back as 1937, Sir Geoffrey Keynes was advocating local excision and radiotherapy as a means of treatment for primary breast cancer. Over the last 10 years or so there has been a renewed interest in this approach, and many groups in France, Canada, the United States, and the United Kingdom have published series of data from uncontrolled studies suggesting that the outcome for breast conservation is equivalent to that following mastectomy for breast cancer. Two recently published controlled randomized trials comparing mastectomy and radiotherapy with local excision and radiotherapy, from Guy's Hospital, London, and from the Tumour Institute in Milan (Atkins, Haward, Klugman, & Wayte, 1982; Veronesi, Saccozzi, & Dei Vecchio, 1981) have suggested that, at least for the stage I lesions under the size of 2 cm, the outcomes in survival and local control are identical, albeit with the relatively short follow-up possible to date. For these reasons there has been a recent shift in fashion detectable in this country toward more and more conservative approaches, while at the same time the Cancer Research Campaign has recently launched a randomized controlled trial throughout the United Kingdom to compare mastectomy and breast conservation for all "operable" cases of breast cancer. We may yet look forward to the day when mastectomy becomes an obsolete procedure, but unfortunately we are still a long way from realizing the other ambition, which is to increase the cure rate of this all too common disease. The hard fact remains that, irrespective of local therapy, only about 30 percent of the most favorable cases can be considered cured, as judged by survival beyond 20 years (Brinkley & Haybittle, 1975).

Adjuvant Systemic Therapy

In about 70 percent of women subjected to mastectomy for apparently localized cancer of the breast, blood borne dissemination of cancer cells has already occurred, and these can multiply to form secondary growths. Untreated, they progress, and will contribute to the death of the patient up to 20 years after surgery. It would seem reasonable, therefore, to hope that some form of treatment directed at the elimination of the micrometastases would lead to an improvement in survival following local treatment for "early" carcinoma of the breast. This is referred to as *adjuvant systemic therapy*, and the treatment used can be endocrine agents or anticancer drugs. Because all such treatments have unwanted side effects, it is generally accepted that some form of selection is necessary to predict that group women most likely to develop distant metastases. Most clinicians would now agree that trials of toxic systemic therapy should concentrate on the node-positive group of patients following mastectomy but, where the systemic therapy is relatively free of short-term or long-term side effects, then perhaps all women with operable breast cancer might be considered for such complementary therapy. This subject has now become highly controversial. Initial encouraging results following the use of adjuvant chemotherapy have encouraged most American clinicians to use this treatment as a routine in all patients with involvement of axillary nodes following mastectomy. However, the regimens used are toxic in the short term (their long-term sequelae are as yet uncertain), and because of this the majority of British clinicians consider the treatment to be still highly experimental. In contrast, there is greater enthusiasm for adjuvant *endocrine* therapy in the United Kingdom because of its relative lack of toxicity, whereas in the United States, if endocrine agents are used at all, they are used in combination with the cytotoxic drugs.

The Management of Advanced Breast Cancer

The majority of women with locally advanced breast cancer not treatable by mastectomy will be dead within five years, and the majority of women with distant metastases will be dead within two years. For this reason, treatment for these patients is directed primarily at palliation. Locally advanced disease can often be controlled by radiotherapy, which again can be used for painful bone secondaries. Apart from symptomatic control, temporary regression of these lesions can be achieved in a significant proportion of cases by the use of endocrine or chemotherapeutic approaches. Approximately 30 percent of breast cancers retain receptor mechanisms that make the cells responsive to endocrine control mechanisms. For this reason, approximately one-third of premenopausal women with breast cancer will respond to oophorectomy, and a similar proportion of postmenopausal women will respond to antiestrogen therapy with such agents as tamoxifen. Occasionally, these responses are prolonged and can produce a worthwhile symptom-free extension to the patient's life. Treatment with combinations of cytotoxic drugs may produce objective responses in up to 70 percent of all patients with advanced breast cancer. These responses, unfortunately, rarely extend beyond 18 months and are associated with serious side effects, such as nausea, vomiting, alopecia, cystitis and bowel disturbance. Although widely used in the United States, they tend to be advocated as second-line therapy in the United Kingdom, or on occasions to rescue the patient from a life-threatening complication of the disease. To date there is little evidence that either endocrine therapy or chemotherapy produce a *significant* prolongation of life compared with symptomatic control alone, for patients in general, even though objective regressions of the disease may occur in some cases. However, in the future, with a more rational selection of therapy based on biological characteristics of the tumor, such as the presence or absence of estradiol receptors, or in vitro cytotoxic sensitivity tests, it may be possible to improve these results.

The Public Image of Cancer

The pattern of illness in our society has changed over time. During the last three centuries the proportion of deaths accounted for by the infectious diseases, such as tuberculosis, bronchitis, pneumonia, and influenza, has declined. Deaths due to noninfectious conditions, such as pregnancy and diseases of infancy, have shown a similar trend, but they have done so to a lesser extent, and heart disease and cancer stand out as the exceptions. The number of deaths from cancer has, indeed, apparently increased over time.* With these changes in the relative incidence of different illnesses, there have been corresponding changes in the pattern of illness awareness. In the public mind, scourges of the past, such as tuberculosis, scarlet fever, and diphtheria, have lost much of their awesomeness, while heart disease and cancer have taken on this role in their place, and today they are seen as *the* major threats to health.

Lay beliefs about cancer are rather vague, and views about illnesses in general are not only incomplete but also incorporate inaccuracies and misconceptions. At the level of the body itself, people have a fairly poor awareness of the organs and their functions. In a study by Boyle (1970), it was found that the majority of a lay sample could not correctly locate the stomach, the heart, the kidneys, and the liver. Nor was there much agreement between this sample and a group of physicians in the definition of commonly used medical terms. In a more recent study, male and female patients awaiting abdominal surgery similarly were asked about the location and functions of various bodily organs (Pearson & Dudley, 1982). Not only were the patients interviewed generally unaware of these, but the interviews showed many active misconstruals. Of the sample of 81 patients, 10 believed the duodenum to be the name of an ulcer, instead of a functional part of the gastrointestinal tract; 11 patients thought they had two livers, one on each side of the body; and 15 thought that the gallbladder is concerned with the urine, or located it in the pelvic area. Such ignorance seems fairly widespread. It is not limited to the less well-educated, and this is demonstrated in a study by Blum (1977), who asked undergraduate and graduate college students to outline the body and draw and label the internal organs. Of those who included the heart, 11 percent misplaced it; the liver was included by a minority only, and 57 percent of these put it in the wrong place. Such findings have important implications for people's knowledge about illness, since they will obviously have difficulty in understanding disease processes if they are unfamiliar with the anatomical structures and physiological functions that they involve.

Furthermore, cancer has perhaps a greater potential to confuse than many other conditions because of the umbrella nature of the term. The same word, or its alternative, malignancy, is used to describe conditions with very different kinds of symptoms. It can refer to a generalized condition, such as of the blood stream in leukemia, or to the disease of various specific organs. Also, it is used to refer both to cases of primary disease, where there may be few if any symptoms and little if any discomfort, and to cases of secondary or disseminated disease, where symptoms may be multiple and severe. Thus while medical opinion may prefer to regard *cancer* as a summary label covering a family of related diseases with varied implications, it nevertheless evokes a generalized image for the layperson. This image is not a favorable one. Wyler, Masuda, and Homes (1968) asked subjects to rate 126 diseases for their seriousness, and found that

---

*Statistics must be treated cautiously, and this does not necessarily mean that there has been an increase in the actual incidence of the disease. An alternative interpretation could be that cancer has merely become more fairly represented in the statistics, as medical interest has grown and methods of diagnosis have become more sophisticated.

leukemia and cancer were ranked first and second respectively. In another study, a semantic differential technique was used to determine attitudes to cancer, tuberculosis, polio, and mental illness (Jenkins, 1966). Cancer was the illness that people most often associated with a high incidence, with death, and with pain. It emerged as the most talked about and thought about of the diseases and yet, almost paradoxically, was considered to be the most mysterious. It was also rated as the most "powerful" and difficult to prevent, and subjects showed a more helpless and fatalistic attitude toward cancer than toward any of the other three illnesses with which it was compared.

Among the best known surveys of attitudes and beliefs about cancer are those of the Manchester Regional Committee on Cancer. Repeated studies have been carried out as part of an educational program, to provide base-line data and indices of change in the target communities (Paterson & Aitken-Swan, 1958; Briggs & Wakefield, 1966; Knopf, 1974). In the 1966 survey, 59 percent of the sample reported that cancer kills more people than any other disease, and it was seen as more alarming than heart disease, mental disease, bronchitis, and tuberculosis. Only 67 percent thought it was to some extent curable. Almost 90 percent recognized the value of early treatment, and most were aware of the possible seriousness of a breast lump, giving cancer as the first or second explanation of this symptom. A variety of factors were listed as possible causes of cancer. Two of those most commonly cited were knocks and smoking, but heredity, infections, and an "immoral life" were also frequently mentioned. A straight comparison between this survey and that of 1974 is problematic, since there are some differences in the composition of the two samples. Nevertheless, it seems that over this time there may have been a marginal decline in the alarm associated with cancer, and some increase in optimism. Nearly 75 percent at this later date believed that cancer was to some extent curable, and 54 percent had heard of somebody being cured of cancer. In the earlier study, the percentages were 67 and 44 percent respectively. There was also an increased appreciation of factors other than cancer as possible causes of a lump in the breast. In neither survey were opinions evenly distributed over the population; older women and those with poorer socioeconomic backgrounds were less well-informed, more pessimistic, and held more mistaken beliefs. It was in the lower socioeconomic classes, in particular, that the changes in awareness over time seemed to have occurred.

Another important survey is that undertaken by the American Cancer Society, in this case focusing specifically on breast cancer. The sample as a whole had a relatively optimistic view of probable outcome. Of these 34 percent thought that most people with breast cancer would survive, and another 27 percent estimated the survival rate at 50 percent. There was an exaggerated view of the prevalence of the disease; 56 percent estimated this at 10 percent or more, and 38 percent said that breast lumps were cancerous in half or more than half of cases. Also, 62 percent thought that a blow or injury could cause breast cancer, but only a minority recognized the role played by age and a family history of breast cancer in increasing risk. A number of conclusions emerge from these and other surveys.*

*See also Hill et al., 1975; Levine, 1962; Stillman, 1977; Tenovus, 1972; Van den Heuvel, 1977.

1. Cancer is seen as the most alarming and serious of diseases, in spite of the fact that heart disease actually causes more deaths.
2. Judgments of prognosis are not over-pessimistic for the population as a whole; a majority now believe that cancer is curable. Older and lower income groups are more likely than others to believe that cancer can never be cured.
3. Most people know of someone who has had or has cancer. Such contact can incline a person to optimism or pessimism, depending upon the outcome in that particular case.

Summary

Descriptions of breast cancer occur throughout history, and it is today a focus of much concern, with one in 14 women developing the disease at some time during their lives. Most breast cancers are of the invasive adenocarcinoma variety and manifest first as an ill-defined lump. The cancer can then infiltrate locally within the breast and to the axillary lymph nodes in the armpit; the extent of such infiltration determines the clinical stage of the disease. The grade of malignancy can also be assessed, and this is determined by the degree of differentiation of the cancer cells themselves: poorly differentiated cells carry the worst prognosis. Following local invasion, the disease may then spread into the bloodstream, and cells can be deposited in the bones, liver, lungs, or brain.

Within the United Kingdom, the most common surgical treatment is the modified radical mastectomy or a simple mastectomy together with radiotherapy where indicated. In selected cases, some surgeons will perform a local wide excision of the tumor, followed by radiotherapy. Trials are in progress to determine the relative effectiveness of such conservative approaches. Chemotherapy may be used alongside surgery where there is evidence of spread, and it has been suggested that it be used routinely where there is involvement of the axillary nodes. There is some controversy about this, however, because of the toxic effects of the treatment, and endocrine therapy may offer a less toxic alternative. Where the disease is advanced at the time of discovery, radiotherapy can be employed to control symptoms, and chemotherapy or endocrine agents may be administered with the aim of achieving a temporary regression of the disease. In the case of both early and advanced cancers, it is hoped that future research will enable us to select the most suitable therapy for each patient, given the functional and biological profile of their disease.

Laypeople are ready to talk about the implications of cancer as a disease entity, without making the finer distinctions that a more sophisticated medical knowledge would require. The public image of cancer in general is that of a serious and alarming illness, but the majority of people do now believe that cancer is curable in some cases.

2

The Stress of Breast Cancer

A diagnosis of breast cancer is critical in its physical implications, and it is also a crisis for the patient at an emotional level. Ervin (1973) has remarked that "there are few physical conditions which threaten a woman on so many fronts simultaneously" (1973, p. 42). Anxiety, depression, and anger may be triggered by the images that the term *cancer* evokes while, at the same time, the removal of the breast and any other treatment will create additional strains. The multi-faceted threat is one that unfolds over time, from the first discovery of the breast lump, and the woman's experience at any one stage is colored by what has gone before and her reactions to this. The diagnosis of cancer has a different impact on the woman who strongly anticipated this eventuality than on one for whom it seemed a remote possibility; and the final adaptation to the illness and to the mastectomy in later years depends on the woman's earlier reactions and the ways of adapting she chose at that time. In this chapter we consider first the patients' adjustment following mastectomy, with a subsequent discussion of the specific threats and conflicts associated with a diagnosis of cancer and with the loss of the breast. Evidence relating to the psychological impact of lumpectomy is scant, and is referred to in that section. Finally, we address the effects of radiotherapy and systemic therapy.

Adjustment in Mastectomy Patients

The Preoperative Period

Bard and Sutherland (1955) have called the period before surgery the anticipatory phase, when the woman is reacting not so much to what is happening then but to the possible implications of these events for the future. Surveys have shown that the majority of women are aware of an association between breast symptoms and cancer. Most women do indeed experience anxiety before the diagnosis, and Maguire (1976) reported that only 8 percent of his sample claimed not to have been at all concerned at this time. Indeed, in one questionnaire study, 42 percent said that the period immediately after finding the lump was the *most* stressful part of the whole experience (Jamison, Wellisch, & Pasnau, 1978). The procedures that are followed for determining whether or not there is a malignancy vary. Many women now have an outpatient biopsy, and receive feedback about their condition before they go into hospital. Some of these women have anticipated the outcome, and react stoically to the news that they have to have a mastectomy. Others are taken by surprise, and their reaction may be one of shock and horror.

> Patient: He was extremely abrupt and more or less told me on the spot that the whole breast would have to be removed. Which came as a bolt out of the blue because nobody had actually said anything at all, you know. I mean the word *cancer* had never been mentioned at all. He was extremely abrupt, and I was completely unprepared for this. I cried. I walked all around the back streets crying. And that was it; I was just faced with it.

> Patient: He said to me, I always remember it.... Oh I could have.... well, you know, I think I was passing out when he told me. He said "You know that you'll have to come in to have your breast off?" And I just looked at him. I said "No. In fact if I'd known that, then I probably wouldn't have come."

Others have rationally acknowledged the possibility of cancer, but have not emotionally come to terms with it.

> Patient: Although I knew it could have been that, when I heard the doctor say it, it really upset me. I cried and cried. I was like that for a week or more. I cried nearly all the time."

Another practice followed is to excise the lump, and then proceed in a subsequent operation to mastectomy if this is indicated. Here, as with an outpatient biopsy, the patient is aware before the mastectomy that this is the operation she will undergo. Finally, some surgeons perform a *frozen section*, a procedure which has very different psychological implications for the patient. In this case she is admitted directly to the hospital for a single operation, and it is determined in the course of this operation whether or not a mastectomy is required. The patient may have been given some indication beforehand of the likelihood of this outcome, on the basis of the surgeon's clinical examination, but will know this for sure only when she recovers from the general anesthetic. She is thus simultaneously confronted with both the mastectomy and the confirmation of cancer, a confrontation that may be difficult to handle psychologically if she has not adequately prepared herself for it. It has been claimed on this basis, and on the basis of clinical observation, that this procedure causes greater anxiety, but it would be useful to have empirical evidence about the relative impact on patients of different kinds of biopsy.

Hospitalization and surgery may be as terrifying, for some patients, as other concerns. Surgery has been described as "a planned physical assault" on the body (Gruendemann, 1965), although one to which the patient has consented. The threat of the removal of any body part, the separation from family and friends, and the patient's dependency and loss of control, can resurrect earlier fears of loss, separation, and vulnerability (Deutsch, 1942). Most patients, in addition to this general insecurity, experience clearly focused concerns about surviving the anesthetic and about the pain and discomfort to be experienced after surgery (Carnevali, 1966; Ramsay, 1972; Renshaw, 1974). Anxiety levels in general surgical patients have been measured throughout their hospital stay, with the finding that these levels peak on admission (Wilson-Barnett, 1978), and that they are generally higher before than after surgery (Auerbach, 1973; Spielberger, Auerbach, Wadsworth, Dunn, & Taulbee, 1973). Janis (1958) has argued that a moderate degree of anxiety before surgery may be adaptive, and that this reflects a realistic recognition of danger and a rehearsal of responses. According to this model, both low and high levels of anxiety are maladaptive, since the former suggests an unrealistic and overoptimistic expectation of what is entailed, and the latter suggests an exaggerated view of threat and an engulfment by anxiety. Neither of these facilitate the patient's psychological preparation for surgery. Maguire (1976) has similarly suggested that negative reactions immediately after mastectomy are most likely to occur when the patient has either been extremely fearful before surgery or has had unrealistically positive expectations of what would happen.

The Postoperative Period

Although some women feel despair or bitterness after their mastectomy, it seems that only a minority of them see this period as being the most stressful (Jamison et al., 1978). Many women are quite accepting at this time, since the ambiguity has been resolved and the operation itself is behind them.

> Patient: I had an awful dread of not coming round after the anesthetic. I always have. And when I opened my eyes, I knew I was there. I didn't think about anything else at all. I was just there. It was lovely. I didn't care how I felt, what I had to go through at all. It was just great to be alive.

Some patients are positively euphoric, but this extreme reaction is not very stable, and the patient who is euphoric postoperatively may later become depressed (Wabrek & Wabrek, 1976). In the hospital the patient has the support of the nurses and her fellow-patients and does not have to think of the future. However, when she returns home she must face the realities of her situation.

> Patient: I was as happy as a sandboy when I came back from the operation. Well, I knew very well that I'd come back and that was it and I'd got to make the best of it. I was happy enough then. It was when I came home that I felt it! When I came home and was on my own again. But when I was on the ward with all the patients I was fine. I could have stayed there. I really loved it.

After she leaves the hospital, the patient moves toward an adjustment to her illness and to the loss of the breast. This stage is termed the *reparative phase* by

Bard and Sutherland (1955). Many women have difficulty in making the adjustment, and research tends to bear out Renneker and Cutler's early observation that postoperative depression is "a common sequel to mastectomy, and is marked by anxiety, insomnia, depressive attitudes, occasional ideas of suicide, and feelings of shame and worthlessness" (1952, p. 834). Estimates of the incidence of distress reported in the literature are variable. In Downie's questionnaire study (1976), 34 out of 100 women admitted to varying degrees of postoperative depression; in another study, 50 percent admitted to anxiety or depression (Roberts, Furnival, & Forrest, 1972); and Torrie (1970) found that, of 1,400 women contacted, 83 percent had experienced depression in the first year after their operation. Estimates are less variable where researchers have thought in terms of difficulties of "psychiatric" proportions, rather than in terms of a more general and less easily defined concept of distress. Three studies consistently suggest that the incidence of severe anxiety and depression postmastectomy is in the region of 20 to 25 percent, in spite of differences in the methods of assessment that they employed (Maguire, Lee, Bevington, Küchemann, Crabtree, & Cornell, 1978; Morris, Greer, & White, 1977; Worden & Weisman, 1977). In all studies, however, there is a wide range of response *between individuals*, clearly illustrated by the findings of one survey in which 60 percent claimed an excellent emotional adjustment while nearly one-quarter said that they had had thoughts of suicide (Jamison et al., 1970).

There have been few attempts to compare emotional outcomes of mastectomy with those of other illnesses and treatments. Hollander, Gonnella, and Parker (1979) asked a group of cancer "rehabilitation experts" to estimate the typical recovery periods for various functions in mastectomy, laryngectomy, and colostomy patients. The experts felt that psychological adaptation for mastectomy patients would be accomplished relatively quickly, within three months, compared with twelve months for the colostomy and laryngectomy patients. Worden and Weisman (1977) compared breast cancer patients with a group of patients with several kinds of cancer, including Hodgkin's disease, melanoma, and cancer of the colon. They concluded that while "depression, lowered self-esteem, chronic fatigue, persistent health concerns, many physical complaints, and uncertainty about the future do occur in about 20 percent of mastectomy patients . . . the same symptoms happen with about equal frequency in women with other forms of cancer" (1977, p. 74). They conclude, therefore, that mastectomy does not present unique problems of adjustment. Since most forms of cancer involve both a threat to life and fairly aggressive treatment, common difficulties of adjustment would, indeed, be anticipated, although the specific nature of the problems experienced might be different. Thus, for example, in one study women treated for genital cancer were found to have more sexual and marital difficulties than those treated for breast cancer, but the latter reported less self-confidence (Wenderlein, Protzel, & Lehrl, 1979). Worden and Weisman (1977) note that for mastectomy patients the time of greatest emotional vulnerability was at the second follow-up, at about eight to ten weeks, whereas other cancer patients experienced this peak around the time of diagnosis, again indicating differences between patient groups in patterns if not overall extent of difficulty.

Adjustment Over Time

Several studies have followed through the same group of breast cancer patients over time. Morris and colleagues (1977) studied a group of 91 breast cancer patients and 69 controls with benign breast disease over a two-year period. They found that just under one-half of the breast cancer group claimed to be distressed either by the fact of cancer, or by mastectomy, or by both, at three months after surgery. By 12 months this figure had decreased to just over a quarter, and then showed another, but very slight, decrease by the end of the subsequent year. Maguire et al. (1978) studied a group of 75 breast cancer patients and 50 patients with benign breast disease over a one-year period. They noted a fall in depression over this time, with 27 percent of the mastectomy patients showing moderate or severe levels of depression at four months after surgery and 21 percent at 12 months. These findings suggest an improvement over time, but this is not a consistent observation. In Morris' study, patients were compared on the Hamilton rating scale for depression. The number of mastectomees who scored more than 10 on this scale fell from 22 percent, when assessed preoperatively, to 17 percent when assessed three months after surgery, but then later rose to their former level. The figures at 12 months and 24 months follow-up were 23 and 22 percent respectively. Indeed, it was only at the 24 month follow-up that the percentage who were depressed in the mastectomy group was *significantly* higher than that for the benign disease group. Furthermore, in the study by Maguire et al. (1978), although the incidence of depression declined, there was little change in the number showing symptoms of anxiety over time. At the four month follow-up, this number was 21 percent and at 12 months it was 19 percent. These two studies thus provide inconsistent evidence for progressive improvement in emotional status. Other studies have suggested an apparent *deterioration* in adjustment. Polivy (1977) asssessed self-image in mastectomy patients, other patients with benign breast disease, and general surgical controls. She found that total self-image for the former group remained constant from the presurgical assessment until the follow-up from four to six weeks after surgery, but that at the second follow-up at six to eleven months after surgery self-image had significantly worsened. Eisenberg and Goldenberg (1966) similarly reported a worsening in attitude in the 18 months between their first and second assessments postmastectomy, in spite of an improvement in activity status over this time. There is relatively little information available in the literature on longer term adjustment, but again no evidence that initial levels of upset are much altered with time. Ray (1977) compared women who had had a mastectomy from 18 months to five years earlier with a matched group of cholecystectomy patients. The former were found to be significantly less well-adjusted in terms of anxiety and depression, they were more withdrawn, and they tended to have lower self-esteem. Scores on none of these indices varied with time since surgery.

It is at first surprising not to find evidence of a clear pattern of improvement in the first few years after mastectomy. It has already been mentioned that this period has been described as the reparative phase, implying the assumption of just such an improvement. However, distress immediately after mastectomy may be blunted by a state of shock and numbness, with this being followed by a summoning of defenses against anxiety. An apparent deterioration in adjustment may reflect the emergence from shock and the breakdown or abandonment of these defenses, while apparent stability over time might represent the joint outcome of this process together with a parallel development in emotional resources and coping.

Sexual Adjustment

This is a specific area that has been considered separately from that of general emotional recovery. Many women do have problems here, but the majority report no change, and some report an improvement in sexual frequency and satisfaction as an outcome of mastectomy (Wellisch, Jamison, & Pasnau, 1978; Woods, 1975). Morris et al. (1977) found that, at three months postoperatively, 18 percent of the mastectomy patients claimed a deterioration in sexual adjustment. This figure was significantly greater than that for the control patients with benign breast disease. By two years the figure was 32 percent, but that for the benign group had also increased, and the difference between the two groups was no longer significant. Sexual difficulties were most often reported by women of perimenopausal status. In the study by Maguire and colleagues (1978), there was evidence of greater sexual difficulty. At four months, 40 percent of the cancer patients had moderate or severe problems, compared with only 12 percent in the benign control group, and at one year the figures were 33 and 8 percent respectively. Before surgery, only 8 percent in both groups had had such problems.

Several writers have pointed to the importance of the existing state of the marriage in determining sexual adjustment postoperatively. In one sample, 36 percent of the patients' sexual partners claimed that the mastectomy had had a bad influence on the sexual relationship, 57 percent that it had had no influence, and 7 percent said that the influence had been one for the better; those who attributed a less negative influence to the mastectomy tended to be those who valued the relationship most (Wellisch et al. 1978). The sample in this particular study was highly selective, and perhaps not representative, but the findings support the general assumption that a warm and supportive relationship can withstand the strain of mastectomy and may even be further strengthened by the challenge it presents. On the other hand, when there is a lack of communication and support within the marriage, mastectomy adds to the tension and may trigger a further deterioration in the sexual relationship where this was initially problematic. For a broad discussion of variables that might influence the impact of breast cancer on sexual functioning, see Bransfield (1982).

The Threat of Cancer

A Common Stereotype

When people are invited to talk about cancer and the feelings that it evokes, a number of dominant themes emerge (Ray & Fisher, 1982). First and foremost among these themes is the fear of *death*, as either an inevitable or a possible outcome of cancer. This theme is elaborated in terms of the *pain* and *suffering* that is thought by many to be a necessary part of the process of dying from cancer, and in terms of the *weakening and loss of dignity* that people also associate with this process. Second, cancer is regarded with abhorrence because of its *invasiveness*. People describe the disease as similar to a "tree spreading its branches," or refer to it as "eating you away." A third theme is that of the *uncertainty* associated with the disease, and this itself is a content of the stereotype. Few have much knowledge of cancer and its implications, and they recognize that this is not just their personal ignorance. Cancer is regarded as an unknown, even to the experts in the field, and this professional lack of knowledge of cancer and not just the fact of personal ignorance is particularly threatening. Ignorance in turn produces feelings of *helplessness* and *vulnerability*. The causes of cancer are obscure, and there is little one can do to avoid or predict its onset. It comes "like a bolt from the blue," and people find especially worrying the thought that they could already have the disease without being aware of it. Finally, an important aspect of people's feelings about cancer comprises the *conflicts and ambivalences* that it creates. People express inconsistent attitudes and are often aware of this inconsistency. It is in part a reflection of personal ignorance, but it also represents a conflict between what the person thinks he or she knows rationally and what, on the other hand, the person subjectively feels. For example, the same person might profess a strong faith in the achievements of medicine, including the treatment of cancer among these, and yet at the same time feel that cancer is all powerful and synonymous with death.

The Diagnosis of Cancer

The diagnosis of cancer has been graphically described as an "informational crisis" (Shands, 1966). The patient brings to bear on her own personal situation all that she knows or thinks that she knows about the disease and its implications, recognizing her own mortality, revising assumptions and expectations that she has previously held about the course of her life, and confronting the uncertainty and ambivalences generally associated with the illness. The patient who has been treated may regard her own case in the light of a general stereotype of cancer as incurable.

> Patient: I'm not a child. I know there's no cure for cancer. Nobody can tell me. So far as I know, no matter where it is, if it's cancer, we know the result, we know the end of it. So that's all.

Other patients will, however, distinguish between cancer in general and their own particular illness.

> Patient: When it's a lump in your breast you can detect it and do something about it quickly. Whereas the other (internal kind) you can't. You can't always.

> Patient: In the inside, the growth can come back, see. But with the breast, if it's a breast . . . we have to be thankful that as long as it hasn't gone further, you're all right. I think so.

However, while patients often argue that breast cancer is less threatening than other cancers because it is detectable at an early stage and more easily treated by surgery, their arguments do not always carry the full force of conviction. Indeed, only a few see the issue as clear-cut, with either the prospect of an unavoidable recurrence or that of a definite cure. For most, a key element of the informational crisis of cancer is that they do not know what the outcome will be. They do not know whether their previous assumptions and expectations for health and longevity are valid or invalid. Thus, the patient has to come to terms not so much with death as with the unpredictability of the future and with the ambiguity of her current status. She is neither clearly ill nor clearly healthy; her status is one of "at risk" (Baric, 1969). A feature of this at risk role is that even the most optimistic patient may be alert for symptoms that could mean that the disease has recurred. Headaches, insomnia, irritability, weight loss, or general aches and pains can lead to alarm or cause nagging worries. In one patient's words, "You listen to every little pain you've got." Another characteristic of the state of being at risk is that, in the absence of positive feedback signaling a recurrence, it has an indefinite time span. An absence of symptoms does not necessarily mean that the patient has no cancer and, at best, indicates merely that she is healthy for the present.

One question that has often been raised is that of the relative impact of the threat of cancer compared with that of the loss of the breast. This is difficult to assess empirically, given the reticence that some women show when talking about cancer, and the reluctance of interviewers to probe deeply in this area for fear of increasing anxiety. Moreover, the answer depends on the extent to which patients are actually aware of their cancer. Both those who remain completely unaware of their diagnosis *and* those who have been encouraged to deal openly and frankly with the issue and to talk about their fears might feel less anxious. Maguire's findings suggest that it is cancer that is the primary concern (1976). Before biopsy, 55 percent of this sample of women related their fears to a possibility of cancer, while only 18 percent gave the loss of the breast as a main or subsidiary reason for their fear. Postoperatively, cancer still seemed to be the major cause of distress, although at this stage a somewhat greater number attributed their concern primarily to the loss of the breast. Weisman and Worden (1976) have similarly reported that in the first 100 days the predominant concern of the cancer patient is with life and death. In contrast, Katz has claimed that the loss of the breast is the more threatening aspect of the woman's situation before biopsy (Katz, Weiner, Gallagher, & Hellman, 1970) and in Morris's study, at interviews three and 12 months after surgery, a higher percentage claimed to be distressed by their disfigurement than to be distressed by the cancer (Morris et al., 1977). Some writers have suggested that the concern that is dominant depends on the stage after surgery at which the assessment is made. Renneker and Cutler argued that "the original trauma . . . most often occurs on the level of the woman's realization that her femininity is endangered. It is, of course, immediately mixed with the concept of cancer, but this does not emerge as the central problem of adjustment until later, after she has become accustomed to the inevitability of mutilation and managed to attain some sort of psychological adjustment to her new physical self" (1952, p. 834). Age has also been regarded as a factor, with the suggestion that the loss of the breast causes greater problems for menopausal or premenopausal women. Others have argued that this question can only be resolved in the individual case, with the significance of both the illness and the loss of the breast being determined by their specific meaning within the context of that person's life style, attitudes, and values (Bard & Sutherland, 1955). Given the inconsistency of statements such as those above, aiming at a general conclusion, this recommendation seems to be a sensible one.

The Loss of the Breast

This is the second aspect of the "dual psychological conflict" of breast cancer, referred to by Renneker and Cutler (1952), and the threat implied by the loss of the breast is in itself multifaceted. The breast does not have a well-defined physiological function at the time of life when a woman is most at risk from breast cancer, but its loss can cause difficulties of adjustment at a number of other levels. It can affect the woman's body image, her perception of her identity as a woman, her social image and the way in which she presents herself to others, and her marital or other sexual relationships.

Body Image

For some women, the primary image is that of themselves when dressed. They focus on the look of their body as presented to the outside world and, with a prosthesis that matches the remaining breast in size and shape and that feels the same to them as the original breast, the image that they have of themselves may well be restored. Others, however, regard not only their surface appearance as important but think also of the form which underlies it, and for these women the image they have of their body is radically changed following mastectomy, however satisfactory the prosthesis. One of the major features of the body that we take for granted is its symmetry. While there are minor imbalances that we might not even notice, generally speaking each side of the body is a mirror image of the other. This applies to the breasts as well as to the legs or arms, and indeed breasts are often referred to as the *bust* or the *bosom*, as though it were difficult to talk about or to conceive of one breast apart from the other. Thus, it is not just the absence of a breast but the asymmetry that this produces that many women find disquieting in their appearance after mastectomy. They feel literally deformed, and even "freakish." To add to her problems, the woman who feels concern may at the same time feel guilt because of the "vanity" that her concern implies. Within this culture, physical attractiveness is highly valued and yet, when women themselves appear to value their attractiveness, they run the risk of being thought narcissistic or vain. The patient may feel, therefore, that while it might be permissible to mourn for the loss of a functioning body part, grief at having lost a breast is not really justified and is something in itself to be ashamed of.

> Patient: I don't know why (I feel this way). I suppose it's not very important to lose a breast. It's not like losing a limb, you know, an arm or a leg or anything like that. And sometimes I feel very sorry for thinking . . . . I ought to be thankful really that it wasn't my arm or my leg. That's what I mean. And I'm ungrateful and I should be grateful.

Feminine Identity

Mead has argued that the breast is the primary source of a woman's identification with the feminine role (1949), and Renneker and Cutler have similarly claimed that "the breast is the emotional symbol of the woman's pride in her sexuality and her motherliness. To threaten the breast is to shake the very core of her feminine identification" (1952, p. 834). This is something that women themselves find hard to articulate, and patients commonly talk of feeling "less of a woman" or "only half a woman." While the breast does not produce life, as in the case of the womb, it fosters that life and has itself become a symbol of the maternal role. Not only is it part of the woman's maternal identity in relation to children, but in relation to all those who depend on her for care. The soft-breasted woman is one who, according to the stereotype, can be appealed to for comfort and reassurance, and the breast is a symbol of tenderness and motherliness even within the relationship between a woman and her husband. The second symbolic aspect of the breast, its sexual significance, refers not just to its immediate role in any sexual activity, but to the contribution it makes to the woman's sense of her sexual attractiveness to others and of her own sexuality. Following mastectomy, a woman may feel that she is unattractive to her husband or to other men, and that she is in some way a "neuter." Furthermore, while the breasts themselves have a special sexual significance within our culture, the integrity of the body in general plays a role in defining people's image of themselves as man or woman. A disfigured or disabled body can be regarded by some as a disqualifier for a full sexual role, regardless of the specific nature of the disfigurement or disability.

Social Image and Presentation of Self

Whatever their attitude toward their nakedness in private, most women are inhibited about changing in public or showing their mastectomy scar to others and do their utmost to look normal in public. This can mean changing their style of dress, wearing looser clothing and higher necklines, and avoiding sleeveless tops or swimsuits. Occasionally a woman may claim not to care about how she appears now to others, but the vast majority want to have a prosthesis that fits well and provides a match with the other breast, so that their disfigurement is not apparent and they can look "nice." Self-consciousness is a problem for many. There may be a feeling that other people might notice the asymmetry.

> Patient: They can't see, but it's the feeling you have that people *can* see and might say "There's a freak there."

Mastectomy does not physically impose any limitations on a woman's social life, but the woman may become more withdrawn if she feels embarrassed by the fact of others knowing about her operation, even if it is accepted that the difference is not outwardly noticeable. She may feel that her image and identity has changed in their eyes, the image they have of her body and her identity as a woman, and that they are treating her differently. Others' behavior may indeed change. People often respond with ambivalence to illness or disfigurement, avoiding the victim or treating her with pity or false cheerfulness, and this can provide a very real incentive for social withdrawal (Dunkel-Schetter & Wortman, 1982).

The woman who does not withdraw may develop strategies for managing people's attitudes. She may try to act as normal and to mask her own uneasiness in order to set them at ease. Alternatively, she may explicitly draw attention to the loss of the breast to preempt their pity and concern. Instead of treating this as taboo, she may talk openly of her experiences and even joke about the disfigurement.

> Patient: Me, now I have a little laugh and a joke about it. I turn it to my advantage and laugh and joke over it, see.

> Patient: Funnily enough, with the people I know, I usually joke about it. If there is something, some discussion about breasts, I usually make a big joke of it. They laugh at it, and everybody laughs at it. Then I go home and think, well, it's not really funny. I don't find it funny inside myself.

A contrasting way of dealing with social embarrassment is to conceal the fact of the mastectomy altogether. Since the loss of the breast is, or should be, invisible when dressed, there is the option of not disclosing it. Her husband and family and close friends may inevitably have to know, but the option is a real one in the case of acquaintances and new social contacts. The disadvantage of this strategy is that embarrassment may be more acute if and when disclosure does occur, and the woman may have to live her life as though in possession of a guilty secret that could at any time be revealed.

Intimate Relationships

Most women are concerned at the time of mastectomy with what their husbands' reactions will be. They report that husbands can often be reassuring, persuading them of their continued love in spite of an altered appearance, or minimizing the negative effects of the disfigurement by comparing it with the alternative of a progressive illness. Some women try to protect both their own and their husband's feelings by hiding the scar, and not allowing themselves to be seen naked, and there are some couples where the woman's changed appearance is not openly mentioned between them. The woman and her husband must evolve a way of dealing with the disfigurement, a way that takes into account the sensibilities and desires of each, although one partner may take more of the initiative or establish greater control in deciding this.

In instances when the couple's sex life is adversely affected by the loss of the breast, this may be because of the wife's feelings, the husband's feelings, or both. Sometimes a woman experiences a loss of sex drive, or a "blocking" because of negative feelings about her own body.

> Patient: We don't bother now. We just don't. We tried for a bit, but I've rejected him so often that he just doesn't bother now. . . . It's definitely my fault, I know, not my husband's.

Alternatively, she may be concerned about how she now appears to her husband. He may disclaim any concern about the disfigurement and want to resume their normal sexual relationship, but the woman may feel that he cares more than he is willing to admit.

Patient: Personally I don't care about losing a breast, but I have this feeling that my
husband does to some extent. Although he doesn't come out and say it.
They try to save your feelings, don't they? But I have a deep feeling that
he's not very happy about it.

Special problems are involved for the woman who is neither married nor in a
stable relationship. She may feel that a sexual relationship is no longer a possibility for the future and that no man would now find her acceptable. The fact of
having had a mastectomy may discourage her from even embarking on any new
relationship, because of the embarrassment that would be involved in first telling
her partner, and the fear that he would then reject her.

Patient: The only thing is I'm always shy of ever meeting another man, you know.
and I think . . . this comes up in front of me every time and I think "Oh,
horrible, I've got this disfigurement. No!" Mind you, I'd love to get married again. I would. But this comes up in front of me every time. And I'm
really a shy person. I'm not a bold person in that respect you know. I'd feel
awfully embarrassed. There *are* very kind, considerate people who'd see
it my way; but if it were somebody you were very fond of, and he didn't
see it your way, you know, it would be awful.

Local Wide Excision (Lumpectomy)

Mastectomy prevails as the key treatment for early breast cancer, so little is as yet
known of the psychological effects of conservative surgery. Sanger and Reznikoff
(1981) have noted a better body image in patients so treated, compared with
mastectomy patients, but no differences in scores on Barron's Scale of Ego
Strength. The significance of this finding is questionable, given that only patients
thought by their surgeons to have adjusted well were referred for inclusion in the
sample. Schain, Edwards, Gorrell, Demoss, Lippman, Gerber, and Lichter
(1983) also found a less negative reaction to the body. In this study, similarly,
there were no apparent differences between the groups in mood states, but these
were assessed via a postal questionnaire, and such measures may not be sufficiently sensitive for variables of this nature. Both studies are limited in terms of
methodology and sample size or composition. Thus, we do not as yet know what
contribution the lesser mutilation involved in conservative procedures makes to
adjustment, and it is imperative that clinical trials focusing on the outcomes of
different procedures on survival should include rigorous measures of psychological outcome alongside other variables. Fortunately, such work is now in progress in the United Kingdom and the United States. In planning such studies, it
should be remembered that the sample of patients who elect to take part in a trial
may exclude those who have strong feelings in favor of one rather than another
treatment, and a simple comparison of those who offer themselves for randomization is not therefore in itself sufficient. Second, the expectations of women
regarding the relative effectiveness of different kinds of treatment must also be
considered. Women who have limited surgery might feel insecure, knowing that
in the past the weight of medical opinion has been in favor of more rather than
less extensive surgery, and increased fears of recurrence could mask any positive
effects derived from cosmetic benefits of this treatment. Finally, where the breast

is conserved, radiotherapy plays a primary role, and this in itself may cause psychological problems, especially in the short term.

Radiotherapy

The patient referred for radiotherapy following surgical treatment encounters a complex of psychological and social problems. First, it is still quite common for "radium treatment" to be stigmatized. In the United Kingdom, at least, radiotherapy has traditionally been provided in a few major centers that, because they predominantly deal with cancer, can be looked on with trepidation by the local community. Almost everyone in the referral area has known of a friend or relative who has gone for "the radium" and has subsequently died. Second, a myth has evolved around the subject of radiotherapy. Rose Kushner (1982) quotes its modern variant, "any mention of damaged nuclear plants or disasters involving radiation is, as a rule, accompanied by information explaining the potential dangers of the invisible rays. Women get scared, but since patients receiving irradiation instead of surgery usually elected to do so with full knowledge that its long-range effects are still unknown, they are inhibited from discussing their fears." One of these irrational fears is that the patient herself may become radioactive and a danger to her family. Other popular myths are that radiotherapy to any part of the body can make the hair fall out, that it is painful, and that it inevitably burns the skin. With modern techniques, radiation burns are usually avoided, although women with sensitive skin may expect transient erythema and desquamation. One belief with greater foundation is that radiotherapy causes exhaustion, nausea, and vomiting, and much of the distress experienced by patients may be linked to this (Silberfarb, Maurer, & Crovthamel, 1980). However, Parsons, Webster, and Dowd (1961) demonstrated that 75 percent of patients exposed to sham radiotherapy developed symptoms of nausea and fatigue, and this suggests that many symptoms may be a function of anxiety produced by the procedure and patients' expectations of its effects. Finally, there is the social inconvenience of radiotherapy, which often involves long distances to travel, particularly if the patient lives in a rural area, since radiotherapy centers are usually situated in the large towns. As treatment is often three times a week for up to six weeks, then the additional expense and fatigue associated with travel, particularly among older women, presents a genuine additional burden.

It is difficult to assess the impact of radiotherapy independent of the life threat following the diagnosis of cancer and the impact of mastectomy. Forester, Kornfield, and Fleiss (1978) attempted to evaluate psychiatric aspects of radiotherapy among 200 patients receiving treatment for a variety of disorders, excluding cancer of the breast. These patients were interviewed at intervals before, during, and after treatment and assessed using the Schedule for Affective Disorders (SADS). Unfortunately, they chose psychiatric patients as controls. The patients receiving radiotherapy had increased scores for depression and anxiety throughout treatment, but similar levels of anorexia, fatigue, and insomnia as the psychiatric control group were found. In addition, the treated patients scored more frequently for social isolation. An interesting and unlooked for finding from this study was that the type of radiotherapy machine influenced the grade of change in affective disorders. The patients treated on the linear accelerator seemed to adapt very well, and scores for depression and anxiety returned to normal toward the end of treatment. In contrast, those patients treated on the betatron, a noisy and somewhat threatening piece of equipment, tended to fare worse. Another relevant study is that of Margolis, Carabell, and Goodman (1983). They interviewed patients who had *chosen* radiotherapy as an alternative to mastectomy and found that these patients seemed well adjusted and grateful for the treatment. Since these patients self-selected for this therapy, they must be considered a biased sample and their reactions may be different from those of the general population. It is likely, in summary, that radiotherapy can have distressing effects, but that these are of short-term duration. The ideal setting for the evaluation of the impact of radiotherapy in addition to mastectomy would have been one of the many reported randomized clinical trials comparing mastectomy alone with mastectomy plus radiotherapy, but these opportunities have been missed.

Adjuvant Systemic Therapy

Most clinicians consider the majority of breast cancer cases, at whatever stage they are discovered, to be systemic, with the outcome following local therapy predetermined by the extent of micrometastases rather than by the nature of the treatment itself. It follows that if we are to make any further impact on survival following local therapy some systemic treatment aimed at mopping up these occult disseminated cancer cells is required. Treatments that are known to cause regression in advanced disease, including cytotoxic chemotherapy and endocrine therapy, might be of value if employed immediately after the mastectomy and for an undefined but prolonged interval thereafter. So plausible is this new model of the disease that many medical oncologists (particularly in the United States) have embarked on such a strategy before awaiting the outcome of properly controlled randomized trials. A large number of these trials are, in fact, in progress around the world, but the results to date are rather confusing. The subject has been reviewed in detail by Baum and Berstock (1982). At best, most of the studies have illustrated a delay in the appearance of metastases, but there is as yet no convincing evidence that survival is prolonged except in some small substrata. The physical and psychological impact of this additional treatment is profound. In the first instance, patients who may have recovered from the mastectomy and are feeling otherwise well are forced to confront the possibility that the disease is not yet cured, while at the same time being subjected to the side effects of toxic treatment. To quote Schain (1978), "this stage is often described by patients as frightening as it involves confrontation of the realization that additional therapeutic efforts are necessary to arrest the disease." The side effects of most of the cytotoxic regimens used include alopecia, nausea and vomiting, bone marrow suppression, bowel disturbance, cystitis, neurotoxicity, and cardiotoxicity.

Sometimes the nausea and vomiting following each treatment is so profound that psychogenic vomiting occurs in anticipation of the next cycle of drugs.

In recent years, a number of attempts have been made to assess the impact of cytoxic drugs on quality of life and on psychological morbidity, using self-assessment rating scales, questionnaires, or independent observations. Palmer, Walsh, McKinna, and Greening (1980) studied 47 patients receiving either single-agent or multiple-agent adjuvant chemotherapy. Of these patients 58 percent reported severe nausea during each course of treatment, while 76 percent of patients complained of severe vomiting, and two patients became conditioned to vomit before treatment was initiated at each cycle. Of the sample, 70 percent suffered sufficient hair loss to warrant the prescription of a wig. When questioned concerning interference with the quality of life, 20 percent claimed that the treatment was unbearable and that they would never go through it again even if their lives were at hazard, while an additional 33 percent claimed that they dreaded the treatment but would be prepared to suffer it again if they felt confident that the treatment would prolong their life. A recent study (Nerenz, Leventhal, Love, and Ringer, 1984) interviewed 120 patients receiving chemotherapy for breast cancer and lymphoma. Patients reported the commonly cited side-effects, and this study is particularly interesting in that it analyzed the association between these and psychological distress. Both tiredness and weakness were highly correlated with distress ratings, while hair loss showed, if anything, a negative relationship. The researchers suggested that symptoms such as tiredness and weakness are commonly attributed to the illness rather than to its treatment, and that patients so affected infer from this that they are deteriorating. Side effects had a greater influence on distress in the lymphoma than in the breast cancer group, and this may be because the latter faced the additional strains of recovery from surgery and adaptation to the loss of breast. A controlled study of psychological morbidity associated with treatment has been provided by Maguire, Tait, Brooke, and Thomas (1980), within the structure of a randomized clinical trial. All patients had previously had a mastectomy and then were randomized to no further treatment, a single-agent chemotherapy, or multiple-agent adjuvant chemotherapy. The latter group received the traditional combination of cyclophosphamide, methotrexate, and 5-fluouracil (CMF). Of the CMF group, 77 percent had anxiety problems, a similar percentage suffered from a depressive state, and 70 percent reported significant sexual problems. The incidence of morbidity was greatly in excess of that experienced by patients treated by mastectomy alone or by those receiving the single-agent adjuvant therapy. The authors concluded that psychological and sexual problems were directly related to the severity of physical toxicity and were concerned that the clinicians were apparently poor at recognizing this physical and psychological morbidity. This suggests that there is probably underreporting of these side effects in most of the trials published concerning the value of adjuvant chemotherapy. In another similarly controlled study, patients treated with mastectomy were randomly allocated to one of three groups: those receiving radiotherapy, those receiving CMF, or those receiving both radiotherapy and CMF (Hughson & Cooper, 1982). There were no significant differences between the groups at 3 and 6 months, but by 13 months the CMF treated groups were showing a marked excess of psychological symptoms, and these symptoms persisted at 24 months, even after the treatment had finished.

Findings such as these must give rise to concern. The treatments are still experimental (UICC document, 1982); their benefits are yet to be demonstrated, while their costs in terms of distressing side effects are apparent. Even if they are found to lengthen survival significantly, their value to the patient cannot be assessed without entering quality of life into the equation. Where cytotoxic drugs are used, patients should be closely monitored for side effects so that these can be countered where possible. Furthermore, it may also be advisable to alert patients to the possibility of their occurrence. It is sometimes argued that this will create a self-fulfilling prophecy. On the other hand, tiredness and weakness in particular may be wrongly interpreted by the patient where she is not expecting these and be taken by her as a sign of the cancer's progression.

Summary

The diagnosis and treatment of breast cancer is a traumatic event for any woman: a significant proportion experience anxiety, depression, and sexual problems, and these effects can be long lasting. The illness itself has a terrifying public image, and the cancer patient has to revise her expectations of the future. Only a few regard themselves as unambiguously cured, and a major threat is the uncertainty associated with the illness. The patient remains in an "at risk" role, faced with the possibility of recurrence even where initial treatment has been apparently effective.

Furthermore, most women with early breast cancer have a mastectomy, and this poses an additional threat to their quality of life. The loss of the breast can have a negative impact on body image, feminine identity, social status, self-presentation, and sexual relationships. We do not as yet know to what extent distress is reduced where surgery is conservative, and must await information from clinical trials currently in progress. Where radiotherapy is offered, this can cause additional difficulties, but it is likely that these are of short-term duration. Chemotherapy, on the other hand, produces quite severe side effects, and there is evidence not only that psychological morbidity is increased by this treatment but that this effect is long lasting. Patients receiving popular combination regimens have more emotional difficulties than other groups, even after the treatment itself is concluded. Such findings are particularly worrying, given the experimental nature of these treatments.

3

Coping with Stress

Ways of Coping: A General Outline

Coping refers to the "things people do to avoid being harmed by life's strains" (Pearlin & Schooler, 1978, p. 2). They try to overcome difficulties and minimize the impact of unpleasant events by using skills and habits that have been developed over a lifetime. Coping implies a goal or purpose, whether or not this is consciously recognized. It is behavior *directed* toward the solution or mitigation of a problem, and the term *coping* should not strictly speaking be used, as it sometimes is, to describe emotional responses that lack this purposive element. Let us consider some general points about the nature of coping before addressing the specific issue of coping with breast cancer.

There are different types of goals involved in coping. Some coping brings about an objective change in the situation, and this has been termed *instrumental coping* (Lazarus & Folkman, 1981; Lazarus & Launier, 1978). However, the perceived meaning of events can also be targets of coping. Even without any objective change in the situation, the person may be able to revise the appraisal of events and circumstances to make these more acceptable. Perceptions can be modified in the direction of "wishful thinking," or underlying values and desires themselves may be changed so that they are less incompatible with the situation as perceived. Thus we can ignore aspects of the situation that are threatening, and withdraw from goals that are in jeopardy. Then, finally, coping may be directed at the emotional reaction itself. Anxiety, anger, or depression interfere with the person's behavior in the situation, and there may be an advantage in tackling these emotions in their own right even when nothing can be done to change outcomes or the way in which they are evaluated.

Both meaning-directed and emotion-directed coping have been described as *palliative*, but their function should not be denigrated. Both instrumental and palliative coping serve to protect the person from distress, and the latter may in many situations be the only possible way in which adaptation can be achieved and psychological equilibrium maintained. Indeed, it is forms of coping that modify meanings and emotions, rather than objective events, that have been most emphasized in the past literature. It is these forms of coping that are primarily reflected in the "defense mechanisms" first proposed by psychoanalytic writers (for example, Freud, 1946), but which, since then, have been very widely adopted by clinicians and researchers in the field of adjustment. Within this psychoanalytic framework the defenses are viewed as mechanisms that protect the ego from conflict, achieving their aim by "deceiving" the self and distorting reality. The most commonly referred to mechanisms include the following:

Repression: inhibiting the awareness and expression of impulses or feelings that would cause anxiety.

Denial: disavowing unwelcome impulses from within or unwelcome facts in the outside world; focusing on the pleasant.

Reaction formation: acting out the opposite of unacceptable feelings.

Displacement: attaching an unacceptable motive or emotion to an alternative object. This can provide some release without the conflict that would be involved in directing the feeling at its original object.

Sublimation: channeling an unacceptable impulse into a socially acceptable behavior.

Rationalization: disguising the true reasons for a behavior; presenting plausible but distorted accounts of beliefs.

Isolation: cutting off unpleasant emotional aspects of a total experience; acknowledging unpleasant ideas, but not the unpleasantness associated with them.

Intellectualization: focusing on abstract ideas or detailed minutiae and adopting an objective and "scientific" attitude toward the situation.

Projection: disowning thoughts and feelings that a person then believes to see others; attributing to others his or her own unacceptable motives.

Regression: acting inappropriately for a person's age; not accepting self-responsibility and turning to others for emotional support.

Suppression: directing awareness away from a conflict, threat, or unpleasant experience.

An alternative approach to the analysis of coping has been to analyze this in terms of general styles or dispositions. One personality dimension that is particularly important in this context is repression-sensitization (Byrne, 1964). Repressors are those people who characteristically take an ostrich-like stance in relation to threat. The significance of the situation is discounted in some way, and the person seeks to maintain his or her present equilibrium rather than to adjust to a new one by simply not recognizing that circumstances have changed. Sensitizers in contrast are open to, and even on the lookout for, unpleasantness. They recognize and focus on threat, and here an attempt is made to find a new equilibrium that does take account of changed circumstances. This dimension is similar to others that have been proposed. Goldstein (1973) talks of avoidance versus coping, and

Lipowski (1970) of minimization versus vigilant focusing. The second relevant personality dimension is locus of control (Rotter, 1966). The person with an external locus of control tends to see their fate as being determined by chance or by powerful others, rather than by their own efforts. The person with an internal locus of control, in contrast, is one who typically sees himself or herself as "holding the reins," with his or her own actions determining outcomes. While both these dimensions have proved useful, in that they predict behavior in many laboratory and natural settings, the character of a given person's coping is not necessarily consistent across either time or situation. It is now widely acknowledged that personality variables such as these indicate only broad tendencies (Magnusson & Endler, 1977). Thus, the same person may be both a repressor and a sensitizer, or have either an external or an internal locus of control, depending on the context.

Studies of Coping in Cancer Patients

The coping strategy most commonly discussed in the cancer literature is denial, and this can take several forms. Patients may fail to draw the obvious conclusion from the evidence of the treatment they are receiving, and avoid taking the opportunity of confirming any suspicions that they have (McIntosh, 1977). Some may even manage to deny the fact of their cancer when this has been communicated to them directly. Alternatively, denial can take the form of an acceptance of the diagnosis but with a refusal to acknowledge its implications (Peck, 1972). Though denial is without doubt a key strategy for dealing with cancer, it may not be quite as prevalent as it sometimes seems. The patient may be thought to be denying when she does not talk in terms of cancer or of the seriousness of her illness, but this does not necessarily mean that she is not thinking in these terms. She may acknowledge them in her own mind but not want to discuss them openly, because everybody else seems to be avoiding the issue or because she is wary of losing emotional control should she voice her thoughts and fears. Renneker and Cutler (1952) claim that "every woman stops talking but does not stop thinking cancer." Furthermore, a patient who seems at one time to be denying the fact of her illness, may at other times seem to acknowledge it. She may seem both to know and not to know about her cancer, with her perspective shifting according to context and circumstance. Weismann (1972) has referred to this state as one of "middle knowledge." The patient can find no stable point of view since neither can accommodate satisfactorily both her own needs and the apparent facts of the situation. In bowing to the former she must repudiate the latter, and vice versa, and her immediate viewpoint depends on which demands are most salient at the time.

Two key studies of coping in breast cancer patients have investigated ego defenses used by women before biopsy, including strategies other than denial. In one of these studies, 30 women were interviewed and their responses assessed for distress, disruption of function, and impairment of defensive reserve (Katz et al.,

1970). In parallel with this qualitative assessment, measures were taken of the level of hydrocortisone in the urine. The latter fell within a low-normal to high-normal range, and the researchers found little sign of defensive breakdown. The patterns of defense employed were described in terms of six basic styles: displacement, for example, where the patient showed an excessive concern for her husband but not for herself; projection, in the form of hostility to the staff or to the interviewer; denial with rationalization; stoicism and fatalism; prayer and faith; and, finally, a style in which several of these defenses were employed simultaneously. The most common strategy was denial with rationalization, that is, adopting the view that all was well and providing justifications for this view. The researchers attributed the apparently good adjustment of patients in their sample to the use of the coping devices described, emphasizing that distress does not automatically follow from exposure to a stressor, but depends on how this is perceived, interpreted, and defended against. Margarey, Todd, and Blizard (1977) interviewed a larger sample of 90 women, and discussed with them their thoughts, feelings, and fantasies about finding a breast symptom and its implications. Their responses were analyzed in terms of a number of ego-defenses, and then related to delay in presenting with the breast symptom. Denial and suppression were found to be positively associated with delay, while intellectualization and isolation were negatively related. A third study that has assessed coping in depth did so on several occasions after mastectomy and defined coping strategies in terms of patients' general attitude toward their illness rather than the traditional ego defenses (Morris et al., 1977). Five strategies were identified: denial, a fighting spirit, stoic acceptance, anxious-depressed acceptance, and an attitude of helplessness and hopelessness. The category of stoic acceptance accounted for over half of the responses obtained, and patients who coped in this way were less likely than others to change the nature of their response over time.

A Coping Schema

If we look at the literature on the response to serious illness in general, rather than reactions to cancer specifically, here also there have been attempts to classify coping according to its general orientation or goal. Verwoerdt (1972) suggests three categories. The first includes those strategies that involve a retreat from threat, and withdrawal and regression are cited as examples. The second type of strategy involves an exclusion of threat, or of its significance, from awareness. Examples are suppression, denial, rationalization and depersonalization. The final category refers to the mastery of threat, and includes strategies such as intellectualization and acceptance of loss. Verwoerdt's analysis is oriented toward cognitive ways of coping with the situation. Lipowski (1970) deals in addition with behavioral coping styles, but the categories he distinguishes are strikingly similar to Verwoerdt's. They are capitulation, characterized by passivity and either a withdrawal from or dependent clinging on others; avoiding, relating to active attempts to get away from the exigencies of the illness; and tackling, or a disposition to adopt an active attitude toward challenges and tasks posed by illness. Capitulation and retreat from threat are behavioral and cognitive coping styles with similar orientations or goals, as are avoiding and exclusion of threat, and tackling and mastery of threat. This kind of broad classification of coping is conceptually attractive, in that it avoids lengthy and relatively unstructured listings of specific strategies.

Ray, Lindop, and Gibson (1982) have described a schema that was evolved to describe the coping strategies of mastectomy and other patients, and which incorporates features of many of the other approaches described but within a structured framework. Six strategies are distinguished, and they are ordered in terms of two dimensions (see Figure 3-1). Both rejection-assertion and minimization-denial are active responses, in that they attempt to manipulate the situation directly or via the person's perception of it, while resignation-helplessness and trust-dependency are responses that are passive in the face of threat. Rejection-assertion, control and resignation-helplessness all acknowledge the existence of threat, while trust-dependency, avoidance and minimization-denial imply a disavowal of its existence. Each of these coping themes represents a qualitatively different appraisal of the situation and of the coper's role within it, and each is described briefly below, with some quotations to illustrate the character of the theme.

Rejection-Assertion

Rejection-assertion is a way of coping that reflects a view of the situation as basically unacceptable. The patient rejects its implications and attempts to revise these to meet her personal needs and desires. Things seem to have moved out of her control, and her response is to redouble her efforts to establish this, whether or not fruitfully. In the context of cancer or the loss of the breast, unfortunately, there may be little that the patient can do to assert her demands over the facts; her attempts at control are often frustrated and lead to bitterness and resentment. This frustration may be directed against others who, she feels, fail to understand her situation or who are responsible, by association rather than in any moral sense, for her dilemma.

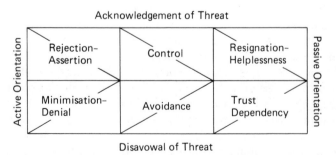

Figure 3-1. Coping themes.

Patient: When I can see there's no help coming my way, then I get really annoyed. And I think that there can be, there is help somewhere. But it's not being dealt with in the right place!

This kind of angry stance may not achieve anything tangible, but it is a very strong one psychologically, and in this may lie an adaptive function where the alternative would be hopelessness and despair.

Control

When control is the coping mechanism, the situation is seen not as a battle but as a challenge, and the patient, rather than rebelling against it, views it as a problem to be managed. She can try to compensate for the loss of the breast and to manage other people's feelings and attitudes. She may also direct her efforts at reducing the chance of reccurrence.

Patient: You just don't lay back (and say) "Oh, I've got cancer, I'm finished," and go moping and everything. The more you fight it the better you'll be. The mind tells you what the body's doing. So if your mind tells your body you're not going to be well, you won't be well.

Or the patient may search actively for information, to provide the basis for monitoring and understanding what is happening to her.

Patient: If I know what I'm up against, I can face it a lot better regardless of how black it is.

Patient: I've been trying to learn as much as I can about cancer so that I'm in the know. My own doctor calls me "Mrs. Know All."

It is this controlling kind of strategy that is often meant by *coping* when the term is used colloquially, in the sense of facing up to and tackling the situation, but not striving beyond the bounds of the possible.

Resignation-Helplessness

The patient who exhibits resignation-helplessness faces the threat, but sees herself as relatively powerless, with events and their outcomes being determined by fate. There is a sense of "what will be will be," and so there is no incentive to struggle against the situation or to attempt to control it.

Patient: I've taken it in my stride. "Well," I thought, "you can't do anything about it. Just go on with life."

Patient: If you're going to die with cancer, you're going to and that's it. But there is no need for the *fear* of it. If you don't accept it, you're going to make yourself worse.

Patient: I must make the best of a bad job. . .what's got to be has to be.

Patient: You've got to learn to take certain things in life. . .if you can change a thing then I believe in grumbling. But if you can't change it, you just accept it.

Trust-Dependency

Trust-dependency is related to resignation in that the patient regards herself as relatively powerless, but events and their outcomes are here seen as being determined not by fate but by other people. She relies on her faith in the physicians and the nursing staff. She is confident because she is in their hands, and in this way she can discount the possibility of real threat or the significance of threat if it does materialize.

> Patient: You must try and understand that everything which can be done is being done for you. And anything that comes will be seen to straight away, no matter what it is.

> Patient: My (surgeon's name) is wonderful; she's really lovely. And she helped...you can talk to her and I know that I'm in her hands, and I'll be all right.

Another important source of external support is prayer and religious faith.

> Patient: I always feel, however much your back is up against the wall, I can always turn to religion. I have somebody other than the doctors to turn to, another line.

Avoidance

With avoidance, the patient acknowledges the existence of the threat, but avoids situations or thoughts that will remind her of it. The threat is neutralized, by withdrawing attention from it.

> Patient: I don't want to think about it. The whole day until I take my bra off in the evening, in the bathroom, I never think about it—that I only have one breast. I don't think about it. I don't want to think about it. I just block it completely out of my mind.

> Patient: I've never looked at myself. You'll think I'm daft. I can't look at myself. In my mind I think it's nothing to worry about (but) I know that if I look at myself I would think "that's cancer." I would frighten myself. You see, I suppose I've got a funny way of looking at it. I like putting my head in the sand. I don't feel like facing things, I suppose.

Minimization-Denial

Finally, with minimization-denial, the patient sees the situation as relatively secure. As far as she is concerned there is little or nothing to worry about and nothing that needs to be done. She may discount the significance of losing a breast for herself and for her husband, perhaps citing her age, her size, the nature of their relationship, etc., as explanations for this point of view. In terms of the cancer, she may dismiss out of hand the possibility of a recurrence of the disease or present rationalizations for an optimistic appraisal.

> Patient: I now live in this absolutely firm belief that all those cancerous tissues have gone away.

Patient: I had no lump . . . not even the doctors could feel it. I must consider myself lucky.

Patient: The lump was terribly, terribly small (the surgeon said). That's what I wanted to hear. That I wasn't going to get it again.

Patient: Even when they were examining me, I had to keep telling them which one it was (because the lump was so small), and the surgeon said to me after, he said, "Oh, I wish everybody was as brave as you. If only we could get people to come when we find it that small, and not let it grow any more." I know I've got some vague recollection of the surgeon coming round and he said to me, "Mrs. X you're cured, you're definitely cured" he said. "There's nothing at all wrong now."

Coping and Adjustment

Coping is directed toward the resolution of difficulties, but it can be effective or ineffective, adaptive or maladaptive, in terms of its outcome. Can ways of coping be used to distinguish those patients who do adjust well from those who do not? First, we can predict that those who have coped unsuccessfully in the past, with the challenges of life as a whole, would be less able to cope with the demands of cancer and mastectomy. High neuroticism and trait anxiety are in fact correlated with adjustment to cancer (Jamison et al., 1978; Morris, 1977; Shonfield, 1980), as are low ego strength, depression, low well-being, pessimism, poor self-esteem and a discrepancy between expectations and actual attainment in life (Cobliner, 1977; Morris et al., 1977; Shonfield, 1980; Sobell & Worden, 1979). General measures of personality, however, make no reference to the nature of the immediate situation and cannot take into account specific factors, and patients who are generally well-adjusted may sometimes react atypically to the threat of cancer and treatment. As Bard and Sutherland have argued, many years ago, "Unfortunately, knowledge of the patient's response to other and totally different situations of stress in the past is not very helpful in understanding or predicting her response to the stress of having cancer of the breast. Each stress experience has a very specific meaning" (1955, p. 670).

It follows that it may be more effective to study patients' reactions to the cancer and to its treatment, rather than their general disposition, if outcomes are to be accurately predicted. One study that has done so assessed patients about to begin radiotherapy for a variety of cancers, and looked at later psychosocial adjustment (Schmale et al., 1982). It was hypothesized that high-risk factors would be extremes of arousal or withdrawal, nonengagement with the physician, and unrealistic expectations of treatment outcome, in whichever direction. Patients were rated for these factors clinically, in the initial interview, on the basis of both verbal and nonverbal behavior. At one and three months later, high-risk patients were found to be less likely to be well-adjusted, with more psychological, social, and somatic problems. An interesting feature of this study is that the reseachers looked, post hoc, at those patients for whom incorrect predictions had been made. They found that these tended to be "quiet" and "minimizing" people who disclaimed problems and talked with little feeling. Some of these, for whom a prediction of later poor adjustment had been made, in fact continued to minimize problems and showed, therefore, good adjustment. Others who, it had been thought, would adjust well, later showed poor adjustment. Not having anticipated difficulties they were perhaps ill-prepared to handle problems when they did arise.

The effectiveness of denial or minimization depends on circumstances. For some vulnerable patients, it may be the only viable response, where the alternative would be fragmentation and despair. Moreover, denial may be benign in certain kinds of situations. Lazarus and Folkman (1984) have argued that, where there is little possibility of controlling the objective threat, then its open acknowledgment may serve little purpose. This is generally true of cancer, and denial may enable the patient to face the future with hope and optimism at little cost. Thus Watson, Greer, Blake, and Shrapnell (1984) found that denial of the diagnosis or the implications was associated with good adjustment, in the short term at least. Where, however, there is something that can be done about the situation, then denial may be maladaptive, and this is the case before diagnosis. Denial is related to delay in consulting about a breast symptom (Margarey et al., 1976), and here it protects the woman from worry but at the cost of depriving her of the incentive to seek advice. Another point to be considered is that denial, since it distorts reality, may be challenged, and a forced confrontation with the implications of the illness could then be overwhelming. One such challenge would be a recurrence of the disease, and we know little of the impact of recurrence on patients who have denied as compared with its impact on others who have openly acknowledged the threat. Haan (1977) and Hamilton (1979) argue that denial can be unstable as a coping strategy and impede long-term adjustment, since it prevents the person from responding flexibly to changes in the situation. Thus, in summary, what is adaptive depends on both the demands of the situation and the needs and resources of the person: "Successful coping requires a balance between what one can accept and confront, and what can harmlessly be ignored or postponed" (Weisman & Worden, 1976; p. 13). Finally, denial, for some people, plays a necessary and integral role in the development of coping over time. A full recognition at an early stage of the reality of the situation may be too costly in emotional terms, and an initial buffer against this may be required to protect the person until other forms of coping can be established.

There is some evidence that coping that is oriented toward control has a positive role in adjustment. Weisman and Worden (1976) noted that "confrontation" was associated with low distress, while suppression, fatalistic submission, social withdrawal, and passivity characterized patients who did less well. Information seeking is one way of establishing control, and a study of coping in patients with four different illnesses, including cancer, showed that this was correlated with less negative effects, in contrast to recourse to wish-fulfilling fantasy (Felton & Revenson, 1984). The latter is an avoidance strategy, and was associated with a poor acceptance of the illness. Taylor, Lichtman, and Wood (1984) failed to find a direct relationship between information seeking and adjustment in breast cancer patients, but they point out that the relationship may be complex with both too little and too much of this strategy being disadvantageous. They did find that well-adjusted patients were likely to believe that they had control over their cancer, and that they had greater faith in others' ability also to control the disease.

This research is still in its infancy, and conclusions are premature. To attempt a summary, nevertheless, adaptive strategies that have been listed in the context of good adjustment to cancer include control-oriented strategies, such as confrontation and information seeking; denial; and trust in others' ability to help. Maladaptive strategies include those oriented toward avoidance, such as suppression and wish-fulfilling fantasy; and strategies oriented toward passive acceptance, such as submission and fatalism. Even if these relationships were to be confirmed, however, there would still be difficulty in assuming that they are causal, that is, that the way in which a person copes determines poor or good adjustment. It may be that certain kinds of adjustment predispose the patient to certain kinds of coping rather than vice versa. Felton and Revenson (1984) have attempted to address this problem, by analyzing the relationships they observed in their study over time, and they concluded that the "unique effects of adjustment on coping proved approximately equal in strength to the unique effects of coping on adjustment. It is thus impossible to infer causal predominance" (p. 350). Thus, a poor initial adjustment may foster maladaptive strategies, which in turn hinder any improvement in adjustment. It must also be emphasized that the optimal strategy depends on the strengths and vulnerabilities of the patient, on the opportunities afforded, and on constraints imposed by the situation with which the patient is attempting to cope. What is adaptive for one person may not be so for another, and what is appropriate in one situation may be inappropriate in a different context.

Summary

Life stresses elicit not only emotional reactions, but also prompt coping. Coping refers to active responses aimed either at minimizing the actual threat by instrumental means or at reducing its impact "palliatively." The latter can in turn be achieved either by a reappraisal of the threat or by a modification of the emotional reaction to it without any change in the objective or subjective situation. The kind of coping attempted is influenced by personality style, and two dimensions of coping that feature prominently in the literature on stress are repression-sensitization and locus of control. The former reflects a disavowal versus an acknowledgment of the threat, and the latter a passive versus an active orientation to coping, whether this is instrumental or palliative in its focus.

There are a variety of ways of coping, applicable to the patient with cancer, and a six-fold schema describing these is presented.

1. Rejection-assertion: reflecting a view of the situation as unacceptable and a violation of the patient's needs and expectations, leading to an active and sometimes hostile attempt to change the threatening circumstances.
2. Control: where the situation is seen as a challenge, and the patient attempts to deal rationally with problems from this perspective.

3. Resignation-helplessness: where the patient again faces the threat but sees herself as relatively powerless, with events and their outcomes being determined by fate.
4. Dependency: reflecting a reliance on others. The patient sees herself as helpless but turns to others, or to God, as a source of support.
5. Avoidance: where the patient basically acknowledges the threat, but avoids situations or thoughts that make this salient for her.
6. Minimization-denial: where the threat is minimized or disavowed.

The relative adaptiveness of specific strategies depends on the objective circumstances and on the person's needs and resources. It is often assumed, for example, that denial is maladaptive, since it distorts reality, but its value depends on the context. Denial can, in some instances, protect the patient against distress, at little cost. Denial can also have an adaptive short-term role, buffering the patient against the initial trauma and providing a respite during which alternative forms of coping can evolve. For some people with limited coping resources, moreover, it may be the only viable response, if they are to continue to lead a normal life and remain emotionally stable. Some ways of coping seem to be empirically related to adjustment, for example, control or confrontation. Such findings should be treated with caution, since it may be that certain levels of distress prompt certain forms of coping rather than vice versa.

4

The Surgeon's Role

It is important to be aware of the stress which confronts the patient with breast cancer, but we must not lose sight of the conflicts and uncertainties to which the surgeon also is exposed. These relate to his abilities to treat the disease itself, the way in which he involves the patient in the treatment, and the extent to which he should and can offer support for the patient in adjusting to her illness.

Controlling and Treating the Disease

In this century, a number of diseases that were once a cause of grave concern have become either preventable or treatable; however, as certain diseases have been brought under control so physicians have had to deal increasingly with others that are less amenable to influence (McKeown, 1976). Effectively, success in one area has redirected attention and effort to areas in which successes are more difficult to achieve. Cancer is one such area. The processes underlying its etiology and development are for the most part obscure, and, generally speaking, there is no immediate prospect of a definitive treatment. This can create a conflict for surgeons and others who treat cancer between, on the one hand, the implicit and idealistic expectations that they and their patients may have of their role and, on the other hand, what they know they can actually achieve.

> Surgeon: I think the thing that hasn't been emphasized is the increasing frustration which many of us feel in deploying treatments which we know are not going to work in a large proportion of cases . . . a lot of what I do is going to prove futile for individual patients. You don't *know* that it's going to be futile, otherwise you wouldn't do it. But you know it may prove to be. It's very unsatisfactory.

Surgeon: What has gone on before may determine outcome. What *you* do may have nothing to do with the outcome. That's not quite true; it will have something to do with it. But the part you most want to do something about— distant, metastic disease—is already determined. That knowledge makes it (pause) less gratifying.

Outcomes are uncertain, and there is even uncertainty for some surgeons about the treatment of choice. In practice they have to make a recommendation and carry this out, but in principle they may have reservations about the relative merits of this and other forms of treatment.

Surgeon: I don't actually offer patients treatment that I feel is best because I don't know what is best. I've no idea. I offer my patients conventional treatment that is being used up and down the country . . . and that's the great dilemma, because I know there are other alternatives, and I don't know whether they are any better than what I'm offering, or worse.

Most surgeons will choose mastectomy as the primary treatment for early disease but, even if they themselves regard this as the best form of treatment in terms of controlling the disease, they may still have reservations about it.

Surgeon: I think mastectomy is probably as distasteful as taking a leg off. It's rather like a failure on your part as a surgeon. You failed to conserve the breast.

Surgeon: I find it a very traumantic operation myself. I dislike doing it; I know when there's a mastectomy on my list I don't feel pleased. I look forward to operating on most lists, but if I have a mastectomy, it destroys my sense of anticipation. I mean, there's no question that I enjoy the sort of operation that involves restoration of function. Those things I see as positive aspects, as sort of creative rewards for surgery. Mastectomy, unfortunately, is an ablative procedure. I don't think it's the answer for treatment of the disease, but it's the only thing we have available at the moment.

Surgeon: I hate doing mastectomy. It is totally disfiguring. The reason is that if it was a curative operation I would feel better. But it is not, and that makes it doubly worse, doesn't it? A loathsome operation.

The frustration and pessimism reflected in the comments above are not shown by all surgeons. While some focus on the discrepancy between what they manage to achieve in practice and what they would like to achieve, and are discouraged by the absence of radical and new developments in ways of thinking about and treating the disease, others are more positive and optimistic. The latter focus instead on present achievements, limited though these may be, and look forward to future advances that allow for the disease to be more effectively controlled. Alternatively, the surgeon may think less about outcomes of treatment and more about the process itself. His concern in this case is focused on following through, diligently and skillfully, the procedures that are appropriate, and, while he hopes for a good outcome, his sense of achievement derives not from this primarily, but from exercising his skills.

Surgeon: For me, most of my satisfaction comes from the technical performance of things to the best of my ability, rather than any sense of outcome. I am

> always pleased to cure somebody, but it is a secondary consideration, distinct from doing my thing, which is surgery.

The surgeon who acknowledges and accepts the limitations of his ability to heal may find it easier to cope personally. Should this view predominate within medicine, however, there would be little incentive to strive for advances in understanding and treating disease. The impetus is more likely to come from a refusal to accept these limitations, whether this is experienced as a challenge and a "positive" movement toward a future goal, or as a feeling of frustration with, and rejection of, the status quo.

Power and Dependency Within the Relationship

The treatment of illness does not take place in a vacuum, but within the framework of the relationship between the patient and the physician responsible for her care. A key aspect of this relationship is its hierarchical nature. The degree of inequality varies depending on the people involved, but the physician inevitably does have the more powerful role. There are a number of bases to his power. He can, first, provide resources that, even if they cannot promise a cure, still offer the patient some hope for return to health. The patient is, in a sense, a supplicant for these resources. Second, within our social system physicians are cast as figures of authority, having the right to make important decisions regarding their patients' welfare, within the constraints of a general ethical code and certain limits prescribed by law. Foucault has suggested that the profession is "invested, at the level of bodily health, with powers similar to those exercised by the clergy over men's souls" (1973, pp. 31-32). Third, the physician has a competence acquired through training and experience that most patients undeniably lack, giving his pronouncements a greater weight than those of any layman. Indeed, this assumption of the physician's expertise is made not only where the issues involved are strictly medical, but is often generalized to others that lie beyond his immediate province. Physicians may be asked for their opinions on social, psychological, or even moral questions, and credited with an expert opinion on them even when they have no formal place in their professional training or experience.

When a patient consults the physician, the latter makes recommendations for action, and the patient is generally regarded as having an obligation to comply with these recommendations. A lack of compliance is regarded as a *failure* to comply, and a large research literature is devoted to the understanding and remedying of this "undesirable" state of affairs (Leventhal, Meyer, & Nerenz, 1980; Ley, 1977). Compliance is less of an issue within the context of hospital-based treatment than where the treatment is self-administered, since the social pressures against a rejection of a recommendation are stronger. It takes more determination to tell a physician outright that you are not going to regard his advice than, say, to accept a prescription and subsequently discard the tablets. Also, hospital-treated illness is generally more serious, and the possible costs of noncompliance in terms of health are, therefore, greater.

Surgeon: The hospital doctor to some extent has power over the patient. Although it's their right to take advice and do what they want with it, most people expect to be dictated to by their doctor and even more so to be dictated to by the hospital doctor.

Surgeon: The hospital doctor says to a patient that he's got some disease, and therefore needs treatment for that disease. And he really must have it. He doesn't really have the choice.

Without this authority the physician would have less prospect of persuading patients to accept treatments whose rationale they do not understand, or treatments that are unpleasant, and from this point of view it can be regarded as a quality to be fostered. It can also be of psychological benefit to the patient, by lifting from her shoulders the responsibility of evaluating courses of action and making decisions, a responsibility that she might not be able to cope with intellectually or emotionally.

Patient: They say, "Right, this is going to be done and we are going to do it," and although you might worry before you get to him, he sort of takes the worry off your shoulders. Once you are in his hands you think, "right, there is nothing else I can do, he's taking over," and you sort of do what they tell you to do. You sort of rely on them really. So they are comforting.

This portrait of a relationship, in which the physician has the authority and the patient is passive and dependent, is one that is conflict-free. It assumes that the perspectives of the physician and patient are compatible, that their roles are complementary, and that the patient is willing to hand over control to the physician in return for his efforts to define and solve her problems (Parsons, 1951). However, although some patients may conform with this model, others are more questioning in the relationship and seek to preserve their autonomy. Friedson (1961) has pointed out that medicine is a specialized subculture, and that the layman and the professional inhabit "separate worlds of experience." While the patient may respect the physician's greater expertise, she may have reservations about how this expertise is being applied to her own particular situation. Her perspective on illness may be very different from his. He applies general rules and categories, and functions as a professional on the basis of his training and experience. The patient, in contrast, is personally involved and brings to her role other aspects of her being (Roth, 1962). Thus, while the physician and patient may agree in the abstract on the ultimate goal of cure, they may have different ways of defining the problem and different ideas about viable solutions. Some consultations can thus involve a struggle for control, from these different perspectives, even though the struggle may be subtly expressed. Its existence is recognized whenever physicians talk of persuading patients to do something for their own good, or of overcoming their resistance, or where patients complain that they have not been sufficiently informed of the facts about their illness and treatment, thus depriving them of the opportunity to make their own judgment.

In the case of breast cancer and mastectomy, the kind of conflict that might arise is one where the surgeon recommends the operation on the basis of its curative potential, while the patient is concerned also with that treatment's personal, social, and sexual implications. Many patients are happy to take their surgeon's advice on trust, assuming that he knows what is best for them. Either they share the surgeon's assumed priority on health and "quantity" of life in decision-making or they believe that he is taking into account their feelings about losing the breast in making his recommendations. At the other extreme, though, there are patients who refuse a mastectomy in spite of being urged to accept it, or who acquiesce with misgivings, because they are not convinced that this is actually the best solution for them. The latter may be resentful and bitter after surgery, never having been truly convinced that the extra safety to be derived from the removal of the breast would compensate for the distress they feel at its loss. Not all surgeons are confident that they can take these kinds of decisions on a woman's behalf. The patient who looks to a surgeon as all-knowledgeable and all-wise may be more of a threat than a support, where he feels that his "world of experience" as a physician does not equip him to take the full burden of this responsibility.

> Surgeon: When the patient actually turns around and asks you what the options are, it's a letout for one, because one's told them and they can do what they like, and you feel it's a bit of weight off your shoulders.

Such surgeons like a patient to participate in the decision-making process. They may hope that she will, in practice, agree to whatever recommendation is made, but would like to feel that this agreement has the force of an *informed* consent.

Both surgeons and patients differ in their preferred stance toward the sharing of information and decisions. Some are more egalitarian than others, and the degree of control actually assumed by the surgeon depends on the patient's behavior as well as his own preference. Control is a negotiable quality, and Roberts (1977), in a hospital-based study, found that physicians permit a symmetrical relationship where the patient is openly egalitarian. However, there are many occasions when patients simply do not feel able to make their needs known. They may consider that their private concerns are peripheral to the consultation, a view that is reinforced where there is little opportunity provided to voice these.

> Patient: Lots of things go through your mind. Then you reject things and say "I can't ask, that's futile, that's silly and I don't want to waste his time."

> Patient: Sometimes you want to ask him something and you forget because he is in such a hurry. I have come out many times from the consulting room and I haven't asked half the things I had to ask, because he looked at me and said, "Sit down on the bed and I will examine you." It takes two minutes, no more than two minutes; and he said "You can dress, good-bye," and he goes out. And that's all. If they would give us a little more time. I think every patient would benefit from it.

Even in a relatively length consultation, the physician may be working to an agenda which is dictated exclusively by *his* concerns. He may ask specific questions that elicit only that information necessary for making a diagnosis or monitoring progress, and the remaining time may be filled by examining the patient, completing records, and making arrangements for tests and treatment. Only the most assertive patients have the determination to interrupt such a routine. For the rest, their needs are not expressed unless the physician invites them to do so and takes the time to listen attentively and to give the impression that he is listening. A belated inquiry of the patient at the end of the consultation, while the physician is writing his notes, is unlikely to be interpreted by the patient as a genuine interest in her concerns and point of view. Finally, a patient may be reluctant to ask questions or challenge decisions because of ignorance about cancer and about her own case. Without *some* knowledge she may not know what questions to ask or where challenges would be appropriate. Thus, ignorance fosters passivity that in turn may reinforce ignorance.

Information: The General Case

There can then be no real discussion of the physician-patient relationship, and of control within that relationship, without considering what the patient is told and understands about her condition and its treatment. Survey after survey has shown that many hospital patients feel that they have been inadequately informed (see Ley & Spelman, 1967; Ley, 1982), and these authors report estimates of the percentage dissatisfied that range from 11 to 65 percent. In general terms, physicians seem to feel that lay people should be well informed about illness. For many conditions, indeed a knowledge of the illness may be a prerequisite for its management, where responsibility for this in part rests with the patient. Diabetes would be one such condition, yet Hulka, Knapper, Cassel, and Mayo (1975) found that diabetics had less knowledge about their illness than their physicians would have wished. So why is it that so many patients are relatively ill-informed? It has been argued that one effect of not giving information is that the physician can then maintain greater control of the consultation; the more knowledgeable the patient, the more likely she is to demand a say in her treatment (Roth, 1962). There are, however, many other possible explanations that do not require the assumption of such unworthy motives. It might be that in some consultations there is not sufficient time to explain to the patient the significance of her symptoms and the rationale of treatment; or failure to provide information might be an oversight, in that the physician believes that others have done so already, or that they would do so at another time; or the giving of information might be postponed because of uncertainty about the diagnosis and the outcome. Alternatively, the physician may think that he has given a very detailed and careful explanation to the patient, only to find little evidence of his efforts at a later date (Ellis, Hopkins, Leitch, & Crofton, 1979). It is the reason for this failure to communicate *effectively*, rather than a failure simply to present information, that has been most extensively investigated. A number of studies have shown that patients remember very little of the information that they have actually been given. Ley and Spelman (1967) found that medical outpatients could recall only 37 to 41 percent of what they had been told within 10 to 30 minutes of seeing the consultant. It does seem, though, that what the patient retains initially after a short interval, is retained over a longer period. Joyce, Caple, Mason, Reynolds, and Matthews (1969) found that patients in a rheumatology clinic forgot about half of the instructional statements made to them and two-thirds of the information relating to diagnosis and treatment, but there was no relationship between loss of information and passage of time.

A key reason for patients failing to remember what they are told is that they do not properly assimilate it in the first place. There are ways in which the patient may be helped to do this, such as by the use of repetition, by making statements that are concrete and specific, and by categorizing information so that the patient knows the significance of what she is being told. Ley and colleagues (cited in Ley, 1977) have shown improvements in both patients' recall and compliance where general practitioners had themselves read a manual that outlined principles such as these. The provision of a brief supplementary booklet may be another means by which information can be conveyed to the patient. It can aid assimilation and recall, even where the information presented is the same in the written as it is in the spoken form (Ellis et al., 1979). Another barrier to assimilation is patients' unfamiliarity with the medical concepts and jargon that are usually employed by physicians in their explanations. As we saw in an earlier chapter, people's understanding of the structures and functions of the body is unsophisticated, and their grasp of even the simplest medical terminology is poor. One study asked hospital patients to define terms in common use in consultations, such as germs, digestion, and malignancy. When these words were placed in simple sentences and the patient asked to define them, the number of accurate definitions offered was very low, with a median of 29 percent (Samora, Saunders, & Larson, 1961). No single word was defined adequately by all the sample, nor did any one subject give an adequate definition of all the words. In such circumstances, it is hardly surprising that communication should fail. Without a basic framework for conceptualization, patients cannot grasp the medical details. What the specialist regards as information, they may experience as meaningless "noise."

> Patient: There's so many medical terms that us people do not understand and when they're talking you think, "I wonder what that's all about, I wonder what they're saying," because it really amazes me when they talk like that. You think "What is that then?" and whatever words they use seem so bad, so long and so bad that it makes you think you've got something really wrong with you, you know?"

To allow the patient to understand, the physician must adjust to her different way of seeing things and frame his explanations from her point of view.

> Surgeon: [it means] putting yourself at the same mental level as your patient. In other words, trying to explain it in a way that the patient will understand, which is very different from the way that we understand it. It is not always easy, and I am sure we don't achieve it, but I think that's the way one at least tries to establish a kind of relationship.

It may, in practice, be difficult for the physician to avoid using medical terminology. He may not be able to express the subleties that he feels are important without employing the concepts that have been developed for this purpose.

Surgeon: Doctors by definition throw the big words at patients. We don't like using the others. We will say 'ulcerative colitis' to the patient rather than trying to define that in non-medical terms, because there aren't any non-medical terms. You can say an inflammation of the lining of the bowel to the patient, but then they say "what's an inflammation?" "Well, it's like you get a boil when it's red and sore" . . . "Oh, then you mean I've got boils in my bowel?" "Well, no, not exactly, it's ulcerative colitis!" You can do your best to bridge the communication gap, but a doctor has learned about ulcerative colitis by reading about it, seeing patients with it, and seeing what happens to them. You can't impart that in fifteen seconds to a patient.

Lacking a medical education and clinical experience, patients attempt to interpret what is said to them from within their own conceptual framework and in terms of their existing knowledge. Information may thus be processed in the light of inappropriate models and assumptions and may become subtly distorted. Much of what patients think they remember can be a *misconstruction* of what they have been told.

It may be important for the physician not only to be aware of the communication gap that exists between himself and his patient, but also the fact that there are more or less appropriate times at which to attempt to bridge this gap. An anxious patient is one who will be less open to novel ideas. In an anxious state, a person can deal only with the familiar and absorb only what she expects to hear.

Surgeon: Sometimes it's obvious when you've made your decision or you are outlining management (that) they're only half listening to you. Because there's such a whirl going on in their minds and they can't assimilate the facts and details. And I find with those patients it's better to make a note when you've seen them, so that you can see them again in a more relaxed atmosphere, when they have had time to digest some of the information. Then to give it to them again.

There are inevitably, however, some cases where the physician faces what seems to be an insurmountable barrier, when he himself cannot enter into the patient's viewpoint nor bring the patient to his way of thinking. Such failures are not necessarily for want of good intentions or effort.

Surgeon: There are some patients who, no matter how hard you try . . . can't understand what's going on. And with those patients one actually ends up with no relationship really. There's very little you can do.

Surgeon: You only give up when they leave your care. I think if you give up trying to make them understand then you've given up the practice of medicine. However, you can quite often see you're not getting anywhere.

Cancer: To Tell or Not to Tell

Within the context of cancer, the issue of informing patients is in fact a controversial one. The question is not just one of how best to give information, but of how full that information should be. Until recently, the majority of physicians were not in favor of telling patients their diagnosis (Fletcher, 1973; Feifel, 1963; Oken, 1961), but it seems that there has been a recent swing in opinion with the majority now favoring a degree of openness (Friedman, 1970; Lancet editorial, 1980; Novack, Plummer, Smith, Ochitil, Morrow, & Bennett, 1979). The climate of opinion varies with time, and there are variations also between cultures: physicians in the United Kingdom are generally more open than their colleagues in the USSR but less open than their colleagues in the USA (Ryan, 1979). Within the same countries, however, there are differences between hospitals and, similarly, differences within the same hospital between individual physicians and medical specializations (Hardy & Hardy, 1979).

In most surveys that have been carried out, the majority of those questioned in the general population say that they would like to be told if they had cancer (Feifel, 1963; Henriques, 1980; Kelly & Friesen, 1950; Lawson, 1980). Would they still want to know if they were actually confronted with the situation, as opposed to considering it hypothetically? That this would be the case is suggested by studies which find that most cancer patients who have been told of their diagnosis say that they were glad to have been told (Aitken-Swan & Easson, 1959; Gilbert & Wangensteen, 1962; Kelly & Friesen, 1950). A somewhat different picture, however, emerges from a study that explored the feelings of cancer patients who had *not* been informed (McIntosh, 1976; 1977). Of this sample of 47 patients, many suspected that they had cancer but only 15 said that they would want confirmation of this diagnosis. How can these inconsistent findings be reconciled? It could well be that patients tend to acquiesce to the conditions of their situation whatever these might be, regarding either knowledge or ignorance as preferable in accordance with the actual state of affairs. It could also be the case that the feedback given to patients in many cases depended on their own initial preferences and the extent to which these were communicated to their physicians. There are, unfortunately, no experimental studies in the literature that have systematically varied communication policy and looked at patients' reactions under these controlled conditions. The issue is therefore one that has not been adequately tackled on an empirical basis.

Protecting the Patient

Physicians are ruled by an ethical obligation to avoid harm-doing and, where information is withheld, justification is usually provided in terms of the distress that an awareness of cancer or of a unfavorable prognosis could cause and the need to protect the patient's peace of mind. To the physician with this viewpoint any other policy might seem like ruthlessness.

Surgeon: I am not all for complete honesty, I must say. I mean, I have worked with people who are completely and ruthlessly honest about things and, having seen that, I think you have got to be aware of the subleties and the human frailties in sensitive people.

Surgeon: I never do anything active to the patient without explaining what I'm doing and why . . . but I don't really explain the nature of the disease. To sit and say what could happen in the future would be horrific wouldn't it? I mean, more than anybody could face.

It can also be argued that to tell the patient that she has cancer can give rise to all sorts of misconceptions about the nature of her own illness, because lay people do not generally realize that *cancer* is an umbrella term. They may apply the single stereotype of a disease that inevitably leads to death, regardless of actual distinctions, so that informing a patient that they have cancer can be seen as risking confusion as well as distress.

Some surgeons assume that patients have a strong suspicion of the fact of their cancer, and that the evidence is there for them if they *wish* to draw the appropriate conclusion.

> Surgeon: I think they understand if they've got cancer. If you say she has a particular lesion, whatever word you use, and then say that you recommend an operation to remove the breast, there can be few other conditions that it could be.

> Surgeon: They may not have heard the word cancer mentioned, but usually they've heard about a lump or a mass, and usually that's cancer to them. I think so anyway. There's been enough publicity about it.

Patients who do not want to know, it can be argued, should be allowed to close their minds to their suspicion, and to leave themselves with the hope that their illness is not serious.

> Surgeon: All patients, well, 99 percent of patients, know if you take their breast off it's cancer . . . but half the patients will not *want* to know that it was cancer, but they know at the back of their minds . . . and they don't want you to say "Your lump was cancer."

Those who do want to know can then confront the physician if they wish for confirmation of their suspicions.

> Surgeon: They usually signal; tell me in a direct or an indirect way that they want to have a chat; they want to know more about the subject. They ask you very directly "Is this a cancer, doctor?" And when you get *very* direct questions like that, one has to say what the truth is, and you have to feel your way so that you don't damage patients with the truth. And yet you don't conceal what they want to know.

> Surgeon: Some of them say, "Well, was it?" You say, "It was malignant; we took your breast off." And they'll say, "Right, were the nodes involved?" You know, because they've read all the books and they're well into it. They want to know and you've just got to tell them the truth.

A further justification for not providing full information is the physician's own uncertainty. To begin with, in the initial consultation, even where he is fairly certain in his own mind of the diagnosis, he may be reticent about saying anything to the patient until the results of the biopsy are received. He may avoid committing himself even to an opinion until absolutely sure.

> Surgeon: If they ask before you've got the pathology [report] you hedge and hedge and hedge. I never tell anyone they've got a tumor, growth or anything until I get that back. That's a personal rule. I've never made a mistake,

but I would hate to make one. You know, to put someone through it and
then have to say "It's alright, it's not cancer."

Then, after the diagnosis, the prognosis becomes the issue, and this too is uncertain in the individual case. Any statement that can be made must be probabilistic.
In these circumstances most physicians adopt a reassuring tone, attempting to
foster optimism rather than pessimism. For example, after the mastectomy, the
patient usually wants to know whether or not the operation was a success which,
in her terms, may mean that she wants to know whether or not she has been
cured. This is a question that cannot be directly answered.

> Surgeon: What they obviously want to know, unfortunately, is the only information
> we can't give. We can never say for sure.

> Surgeon: One says, and one tries to imply that the thing has now been removed.
> Obviously you can't say "Well, we'll have to wait and see. We'll have to
> see. We can't really tell if we have cured you." One tries to be a bit more
> positive than that and say, you know, "Well, as far as we can tell there's
> no sign of it." Those are the words I use and then it's up to them. If they
> are optimists they'll accept it at face value and when in four years' time
> or ten years' time or whatever, if there is a recurrence, they can worry
> about it then. Why worry about it from day one?

It can be argued that the patient may not only fail to be reassured but be alarmed
by a more equivocal statement, even though it might accurately represent the
physician's own uncertainty, because she herself may not be able to grasp the fact
that predictions in the individual case are, of necessity, uncertain.

Disadvantages of Concealment

Concealment may protect the patient from unpleasantness, but it has its counter-
balancing costs. First, it can be very frustrating for the patient who wants information, but finds that her questions are evaded.

> Patient: They're a bit guarded, they don't want to say too much. I always get the
> feeling that if you ask too many questions they wouldn't answer, you
> know. I've tried. That makes me sort of shut up, you know, in a way. You
> know, when I go after four months (at follow-up) I think, "Well, I must
> ask . . . certain questions." And I then ask them about something and
> . . . I just feel that the doctor isn't very keen to go on to answer any other
> questions. I have this sort of feeling that . . . the doctor doesn't want to
> discuss your problems too much with you.

Meeting with evasion, she may speculate about why information is being
withheld, and may conclude that the situation is worse than it actually is.
Similarly, in the absence of open discussion, any overpessimistic misconceptions
that she harbors remain uncorrected. If she is ignorant of the diagnosis or its
implications, on the other hand, this too can have negative effects. She might be
less distressed in the short term, but in the longer term be psychologically more
vulnerable should she discover the facts in some other way: from other medical

or nursing staff, fellow patients, or family and friends. If not from other people, she might acquire the relevant information from magazine articles, or television programs, and the media are now generally very frank in their discussions of cancer. If this happens, she may not only be taken by surprise, but feel cheated and deceived. She may have difficulty in placing further trust in her physician's pronouncements about her case and its treatment, and in relying on his reassurances. The withholding of information thus also affects the quality of the relationship between the physician and the patient. Furthermore, the former has to be on guard not to reveal more than he has decided to tell, and the patient, to the extent that she suspects she has cancer, is also constrained in her behavior. There may be a "conspiracy of silence," with both having the fact of cancer uppermost in their mind but neither feeling able to acknowledge this fact. They may still be communicating about cancer, but in ways that are nonverbal rather than verbal, and in ways that enhance anxiety rather than reassure.

> Surgeon: You get a *folie à deux* situation taking place between the doctor and the patient, in which the nonverbal communication from the doctor is "I'm telling you you must be frightened." This is what comes through to the patient who says, nonverbally, "You're absolutely right, doctor, I am frightened."

Here the attempted concealment fails to protect the patient and at the cost of undermining a relationship from which she might otherwise derive support.

These considerations are fairly pragmatic in their nature, and there are additional arguments against concealment that rest on general principles. One such is that of the intrinsic desirability of honesty as opposed to lying or concealment, and another that of the patient's right to know. Recently, a greater number of physicians and patients are favoring an egalitarian relationship, in which the latter are treated as "adults." This entails on the one hand that they have an obligation to be responsible with respect to their health and, on the other hand, that they also have certain rights, one of which is access to information relevant to their welfare.

Achieving a Balance

Within most of the literature the issue of communicating about cancer is generally regarded as one of "to tell or not to tell," yet in practice the issue is much more complex. There are a range of options concerning the fullness of any information that is conveyed. At one extreme there is a completely frank and open discussion that uses terms such as *cancer* and *malignancy* and presents the facts without any attempt to slant these in a way that is reassuring to the patient. Then, at the other extreme, there is the option of lying outright to the patient and explicitly denying her cancer. However, few physicians would defend either of these extremes. If they tend toward openness, then frankness about the seriousness of the illness might be tempered with a bias toward optimism in their presentation of the facts, and, if they tend toward concealment, this usually involves avoidance with the physician sidestepping discussion about the illness but without actually lying. Most strategies thus involve some kind of a compromise between openness and concealment, with the particular balance achieved being determined by the surgeon's own personal orientation and his perception of the patient's needs. In Renneker and Cutler's words, they try to steer a middle course "between terrifying obscurantism and equally terrifying unabsorbable information" (1952, p. 159), dispelling ignorance without dispelling hope.

> Surgeon: You're always on your guard not to lie and yet not to tell the most awful truth.

> Surgeon: I think lying to patients on the whole is not the right way to go about things. I don't think we have to lie to them. But I think there are some patients who don't benefit from being told the whole truth, every single thing about it. For example, patients who have got a very bad prognosis. Because to my mind that would leave someone without any hope, and I think hope is important as well.

Many surgeons use euphemisms and avoid the terms *cancer* and *malignancy*, and this includes those who wish to communicate to the patient the seriousness of the illness and the possibility that treatment will not effect a cure, as well as surgeons who want to underplay this.

> Surgeon: Not every woman wants to know, likes to hear the word *cancer*. So you try to use other words like *tumor*, *ulcer*, and things. Because cancer is such a terribly emotive word and it has such a wide spectrum of meaning. So on the whole I try to avoid it.

Other surgeons similarly are concerned that the patient might draw a mistaken and overpessimistic conclusion where euphemisms are not employed, but, instead of avoiding the issue, they try to educate her about the meaning and implications of the cancer in her own particular case. They accept that the information they are presenting is threatening, but feel that it can be coped with intellectually, and emotionally, if the physician-patient relationship in the context of which it is presented is a supportive one. To offer this kind of support effectively, of course, the physician himself should be at ease with the subject, not regarding cancer as a symbol of failure and hopelessness but bringing to it the realism and pragmatism that he brings to the consideration of other serious illnesses.

The surgeon's decision is thus rather one of *what* to tell than *how much to tell*. He makes a judgment of which aspects of the situation to discuss, the words to use, and the amount and kind of reassurance to offer. Some surgeons have a policy that they apply somewhat uniformly, regardless of the person with whom they are dealing. This has its advantages. It means that he does not have to make a new decision in the case of each and every patient, and, even more significantly, different members of the same team are less likely to be inconsistent in their interactions with patients if they know, as a general principle, what the latter has been told. On the other hand, patients do differ in their needs and resources. Some prefer not to acknowledge their cancer and its implications, while others choose to confront the threat and to base their coping on this open acknowledgment, and Bard and Sutherland have admitted that "it is doubtful that it will ever

be possible to develop an absolute and infallible plan to apply uniformly in relationship with any cancer patient" (1955, p. 670). In principle the optimal
strategy, therefore, is one that gears the information given to the needs of the
specific patient, but the surgeon should be wary of misleading assumptions. The
old or the poorly educated are not necessarily less in need of information or less
able to cope. Another criterion commonly employed is whether the patient asks,
and the patient who asks outrightly about her illness is more likely to have this
discussed openly and in detail than one who waits for the physician to provide
information. However, this too should be treated with caution as a reliable guide.
Cancer patients often have unanswered queries but do not know how to phrase
these or are too upset to ask (Messerli, Garamendi, & Romano, 1980). Also,
whatever the illness, patients generally seldom take any initiative in a consultation (Pratt, Seligman, & Reader, 1957), and this is especially true of working
class patients, even though their desire for information is no less (Cartwright,
1964). It may be up to the physician, then, to leave space for the patient to make
her needs known, and to prompt her where necessary. Once a dialogue has been
initiated, it becomes possible to "feel one's way": imparting information
gradually and adjusting what is said next on the basis of the patient's reaction to
what has already taken place. This is not an easy task, but it is in principle no
different from many other hypothesis testing procedures with which the clinician
is involved.

Meeting the Patient's Emotional Needs

The surgeon's role in helping patients come to terms with their breast cancer has
been described as a pivotal one (Ervin, 1973; Klein, 1971). It is to him that they
turn, not only with questions about their illness, but also for more general reassurance and support. Some patients, however, feel that this is not forthcoming.

> Patient: You need (them) . . . to show that they do care; that they're not just up in
> that theater [operating room] cutting you about . . . if they could just get
> into their stride of taking more notice of women and how they feel about
> things. If they only did that then women wouldn't be so bad. Once they've
> had a mastectomy they wouldn't feel so bad.

Although it is widely acknowledged in principle that breast cancer causes distress, this may not be dealt with or even detected at a practical level. In a study
of patients attending a breast clinic, Lee and Maguire (1975) noted that patients
signaled this distress, nonverbally if not verbally, but that these cues were not
generally reacted to by the surgeon. Similarly, longer-term and significant emotional difficulties often remain undetected by hospital staff (Maguire, 1976;
Maguire, Tait, Brooke, Thomas, & Sellwood, 1980). Such observations are not
limited to the setting of cancer, and it seems that patients' concerns are not, in
fact, commonly tackled in routine hospital care. For example, Korsch, Freeman,
and Negrete (1971, 1972) have commented on the relative absence of any overt
reference to emotions, in their observations of mother-physician interactions at

a pediatric clinic. The physician's statements were typically emotionally neutral, and were focused on the child's condition, while the mother's feelings and worries were disregarded, even where her nervousness or tension were overtly expressed. Patients also collude in the avoidance of emotional issues; they are aware of the pressures the staff have to deal with and do not want to add to these. The "good patient" is one who is respectful, considerate, does what she is told, and is friendly and unassuming (Anderson, 1973; Morrow, Craytor, Brown, & Fass, 1976; Tagliacozzo & Mauksch, 1972), and many breast cancer patients wish to conform with this stereotype, whether on the ward or in outpatient clinics. They tend to mask their feelings of anxiety or grief (Wabrek & Wabrek, 1976; Waxenberg, 1966), and this makes it difficult for physicians or nurses to identify those who are in need unless they encourage patients to express their concerns.

The degree of emotional support that the surgeon offers to the patient depends in part on the image that he has of his role and its obligations. There are some who look on the surgeon's role as being first and foremost, if not exclusively, one of caring for the patient's physical welfare. They focus on the patient's objective problems rather than her subjective concerns, and they regard her from the point of view of diagnosis and treatment as a "case" rather than as a "person." When dealing with breast cancer, the symptoms the patients have are fairly well-defined and related to a specific, organic disorder, and so lend themselves to standardized procedures of diagnosis and treatment that do not *require* a rapport between the physician and patient if they are to be carried out effectively. In addition, the hospital physican will be unfamiliar with the patient's history and life style, and there may appear to be little basis for anything other than a superficial contact. The context thus encourages an interaction between the physician and the patient that is primarily instrumental and organic in its reference. To attribute this kind of orientation to the physician does not imply that he is not concerned with the patient's needs, but rather that he interprets these in a particular way. He may feel that by adopting this approach he will, himself, be better able to deal with the physical problems; that the patient too will have these as her first concern; and that she will have greater confidence in the physician who "gets on with the job." The alternative orientation, and one which is more difficult to sustain, attempts to deal with the patient at a personal level. Within this framework, the physician is concerned not only with the detection and treatment of the organic problem but with subjective aspects of the illness also. He thinks in terms of the patient's perceptions and concerns, in order to offer the reassurance and support appropriate to these, and this he regards as an integral part of his role in parallel with its technical function.

Surgeon: As doctors we have to be able to manage and cope with all components of the disease, whether they are organic or psychological. To recognize that part of the disease is the psychological reaction to the disease.

Surgeon: I don't think doctors are particularly judged on their performance in technical terms. In fact I *know* they are not. Most patients know very little about the level of skill their doctors have. They admire them for their

ability to reassure them; for their ability to work out with them problems
that may occur in the future; their approachability and their general
demeanor; their kindness, sensitivity, their sense of humor.

There are a number of factors which actively discourage a personal orientation,
leading surgeons to focus on the organic and the objective rather than the
psychological and the subjective. One is the emphasis of their initial training,
which deals with the body and its dysfunctions in isolation from the mind. Then,
as they complete their training and move through the hierarchy from house physician to consultant, so the opportunity for contact with patients decreases and the
initial bias away from a concern with patients' emotional needs is reinforced.

Surgeon: You get more aloof. You must do. You start off as a medical student and
          you are encouraged to get to know the patients you have been allocated,
          and sit beside them and talk to them, and get the feel of it. When you
          become a houseman then you rush around ordering all the tests and get-
          ting everything up to date. You don't have time to sit down and talk to the
          patients for long. You are more concentrated on getting all the tests
          sorted out for the operation or whatever. Then, after, you start taking
          exams, which very finely concentrates your mind on the technical aspects
          of whatever the subject is. And when you come to the hospital at registrar
          level you are concentrating more on the operation or whatever. Then, a
          bit further up, you are headed toward consultant level, when you are even
          more away from the patient and what's happening at the bottom. A con-
          sultant would not be expected by his patients or his colleagues to do
          anything more than kindly inform the patient what is going on.

Another factor is the custom of providing care on a team basis. While one person
may ultimately be responsible for a given patient's treatment, different members
of the team see her on different occasions. This system creates barriers on both
sides, with the physician being unable to identify with a patient as *his* patient,
and thus not feeling the same *personal* involvement in her welfare, and the
patient conversely feeling little sense of a continuing relationship with any of the
physicians whom she has seen. A third constraint is that of work pressure. The
physician may feel that he simply cannot give the time necessary to deal adequately with one patient, given the equally valid claims of others who are waiting
and whose own consultations would be correspondingly shortened. Again, this is
a constraint that patients feel independently and that hinders them from confiding their concerns. If they are to do so, they have to be particularly determined
and well organized.

Surgeon: You often see them with aids—like they will write things down on a piece
          of paper to ask you. Which always strikes me as a failure on our part,
          because if you actually have a discussion that is going to be so quick that
          the patient feels that he has to *itemize* what he wants to ask you. . . .

Yet another barrier to the surgeon's becoming involved with the patient's concerns is the fear that, in dealing with these, he might himself become emotionally
involved. To do his job effectively he must maintain a professional detachment
and not allow his own equilibrium to be disturbed, and one way of ensuring

detachment is to distance himself from the patient. In dealing with cancer there is a danger of the physician's becoming vulnerable to all sorts of negative emotions arising from his own personal anxieties about illness and death, from his sympathy for the patient's dilemma, from his powerlessness in the face of a recurrence of the disease, and from his role in performing a disfiguring operation. Patients themselves can sometimes recognize and sympathize with his dilemma.

> Patient: Maybe that's how he feels about us—that he's got to be impersonal otherwise he is going to get too emotional about it, because he is really defacing us. However we may like it, we are being defaced and he is having to do it.

This is a real problem within medicine: that of caring *for* patients without caring so much *about* them that the physician's own emotional resources are depleted. However, it is a problem with which other professions have also to deal and that has to be tackled explicitly in those situations where a client's distress is the focus of professional concern, as in social work or psychiatry. Here the issue cannot be sidestepped, and helpers "work through" the difficulties and learn to involve themselves with the client's emotions without sharing, or being diminished, by these. It must, though, be acknowledged that in these cases the professionals are to a degree self-selected for their ability to take on this task, whereas physicians in general, and surgeons in particular, may not have clearly envisaged this as part of their role and have chosen their specialization on the basis of very different criteria.

Finally, there are surgeons who like to take a personal orientation, who feel a responsibility to care for patients' emotional needs, and who could themselves cope emotionally with this kind of approach, but in practice lack the interpersonal skills required to do so adequately. They may ask relevant questions and make relevant responses to the patients' statements and enquiries, yet fail to win the patient's confidence at this level. It is not only the verbal dimension of the interaction that is important. The surgeon's ability to reassure, and the patient's willingness to disclose her concerns, depends on his skill in communicating at the nonverbal as well as verbal level. Yet it is only recently that these stylistic aspects of the relationship have been seriously considered within medical practice, and this is an issue that causes some physicians to feel uncomfortable and even threatened. They attach to it the same mystique as patients attach to the more technical aspects of the physician's role.

> Surgeon: There are some doctors who inspire confidence and it's very difficult to put your finger on what it is that they do and others do not. You can see it in your colleagues, you can see it on a ward round when a chap goes round and stands at the end of the bed and there's no rapport at all between him and the customer who's lying in the bed. And the other who somehow establishes that much closer relationship.

The issue of style, for some, has almost a taboo quality. It is seen as something private and individual, and it is not much discussed among colleagues for this reason.

Surgeon: You don't talk with others about their style. Such a question is an intrusion, so some people would consider it. It's a private question about one's personality, a very private thing. Whereas the way that you actually treat a disease, or the way that you do an operation, isn't an attack on one's personality. It's an attack on one's knowledge or skills, but that's more acceptable.

A physician's style, or communication skill, can, in fact, be quite systematically analyzed in terms of nonverbal behaviors such as tone of voice, facial expression, posture, and movements. All of these can communicate something above and beyond the words that are spoken. Here is a very basic example.

Patient: Sometimes he doesn't even condescend to look at you. Sometimes I wonder if they're really listening . . . they are turning away to wash their hands or something. The least they can do is look at you when they talk to you. If they never look at you, if they're flitting about doing something or other, then they're just not interested.

Brief but useful practical guides to appropriate and inappropriate behaviors in the physician-patient consultation can be found in Byrne and Heath (1980) and Cline (1983), and interviewing skills are now taught as part of the curriculum in many medical schools. It is also possible to give students greater insight into the needs of the cancer patient, and to prepare them for their role in dealing with these, by specifically designed courses. Structured opportunities to interview and listen to patients, and seminars and discussion groups, can help to modify students' perceptions of the cancer experience (Cassileth & Egan, 1979), and to increase their empathy (Poole & Sanson-Fisher, 1979). However, such courses can only be expected to succeed if they are given a key role within the curriculum, so that students invest an effort into them and use them to work through their anxieties and defenses. The success of these courses will be jeopardized by any perceived conflict between their focus and the orientation of the course as a whole.

Summary

There are conflicts and uncertainties implicit in the surgeon's role, which can make the treatment of breast cancer stressful for him as well as for the patient. Cancer is a disease that is unpredictable in its outcome, and there is concern about both the effectiveness and acceptability of mastectomy. It is not surprising, then, that some surgeons feel frustrated by the limitations of their role as healers. Against this background, surgeons have to make decisions about the way in which they conduct their relationship with patients. Individual surgeons differ in the degree of control they assume, some adopting an authoritative stance, while others allow a more egalitarian relationship. Related to this is the issue of deciding what to tell the patient about her condition. Patients in medical settings generally are relatively ill-informed, and in the case of cancer some physicians wish actively to withhold information. This can be justified in terms of avoiding unnecessary distress on the part of the patient, but it can have the negative effect of sometimes increasing uncertainty and undermining trust and confidence. It is a policy that can also be challenged in principle, in terms of the patient's right to be dealt with honestly and as a responsible adult. Thus many surgeons attempt to achieve a balance between openness, on the one hand, and avoidance or conceal-ment on the other, by adopting a policy of disclosure that is selective or biased toward reassurance. Finally, the surgeon has the option of relating to the patient primarily in terms of her symptoms and disease or of attempting to meet also her emotional needs. This entails an openness and warmth which some surgeons find difficult to achieve. Two barriers to this more personal orientation are the threat that it implies to maintaining a professional detachment and a lack of training in the interpersonal skills that it requires.

5

Psychological Support: Sources Other than the Surgeon

Counseling and Therapeutic Interventions

The Nurse's Role

Generally speaking, nurses have a more explicit and well-articulated concept of their role than do physicians. This role is often regarded as having two distinct though interwoven aspects: a technical function that corresponds with the case orientation referred to in the context of the surgeon's role, and an expressive function that comprises the kinds of concerns implicit in a personal orientation. The former, the technical function, refers to the instrumental activities the nurse engages in to support the patient's physical treatment and care, and the latter refers to the effort she makes to reduce the patient's emotional tensions. The importance of caring for the total patient, that is for her psychological as well as her physical needs, is very commonly recognized (Brown, 1965; Johnson & Martin, 1965). The nurse informs the patient, reassures her, conveys warmth and interest, and helps to clarify problems and to solve them (Gardner, 1979) but this is to some extent an ideal, as opposed to a description of actual practice. Nurses may want to provide total care, but feel that they do not have the opportunity to do so (Hockey, 1976). Most of the available time may be taken up by physical tasks, and, even if it is not, it is often seen as inappropriate for the nurse to stay by the patient *just* to talk (Stockwell, 1972). Any interaction that does take place, then, usually takes place while the nurse is carrying out some other task. There are problems also in the expectations that patients may have of the nursing role. They sometimes see the nurse as there to care for their physical needs only, however the nurse herself may regard her function, and patients may be reticent about their feelings and reluctant to ask for other kinds of support. Physicians and surgeons too can have expectations that inhibit nurses in their interactions with patients. A nurse may be reluctant to give information and have detailed discussions with patients, for fear of incurring the displeasure and criticism of a physician who regards himself as responsible for what to disclose and what guidance to give (Goodwin & Taylor, 1977; Kalish & Kalish, 1977; Shukin, 1979).

Another problem is that nurses, like physicians, may have emotional difficulties in coping with their role, and these may be greater because of the closer and more extended contact that they have with patients. In caring for the sick, nurses are routinely exposed to anxiety and grief, doubt and uncertainty, and such stresses may be particularly acute when they are working in intensive or critical care units, or with the terminally ill, or even with patients who have early cancer. Cancer has a negative image among nurses, as it does among the rest of the population, with a significant proportion regarding it as the most alarming disease (Elkind, 1978), and some nurses feel greater pessimism about cancer outcomes than is justified by the statistics. For example, Davison (1965) found that, while overall estimates of the curability of breast cancer were fairly accurate, 16 percent of her sample of nurses thought that breast cancer was curable in less than 25 percent of cases. With this kind of perception, it would be difficult to be open and reassuring in dealing with the cancer patient, and many nurses use evasion and a conspiracy of silence as a way of coping with this dilemma (Macleod Clark, 1981). An additional factor in the case of breast cancer is that female nurses can identify with the patient, particularly when the latter is relatively young, so that their own fears of cancer and disfigurement are awakened (Quint, 1963). A natural response in such a situation can be to depersonalize the patient, to distance themself emotionally, and to limit interactions to routine tasks and superficial conversation. This kind of defense may, indeed, be the only realistic option for many nurses, if they are not to experience emotional burn out (Koocher, 1969; Maslach & Jackson, 1982; Rothenberg, 1967). A related issue is that nurses have had no training in counseling as such, and they feel ill-equipped to attempt this (Ray, Grover, & Wisniewski, 1984). Their efforts might even be counter-productive if they were to do so. Their training encourages them to be reassuring and thus perhaps to make light of problems yet, in counseling, a patient's concerns should not be neutralized in this way, but should be talked through so that they can come to terms with their experience. The unskilled counselor may be encouraging a patient to deny or suppress rather than to work through her negative feelings, thus promoting defenses that might in the longer term be maladaptive (Gyllensköld, 1982).

The Specialist Nurse

In the last few years in the United Kingdom a group of nurses have emerged, whose principal responsibility is the counseling of mastectomy patients. The mastectomy counselors follow in the tradition of other specialist roles, such as the stoma therapist, the oncology nurse, and the intensive care nurse specialist. The counselor, acting outside the constraints of the ward routine, can provide a link with the patient's other support services, which include the family practitioner, the appliance officers, and the community-based social services. She can also establish contact with the patient from the time of the diagnosis and maintain contact after she has left the ward, and this continuity of care allows her to deal with problems as they arise and to talk with the patient about her feelings when she is ready to tackle these. At present, routine counseling for mastectomy patients is not available within the majority of hospitals in the United Kingdom, but a service has been developed in Manchester, Edinburgh, the Royal Marsden Hospital (London), and King's College Hospital Medical School.

It may be helpful to describe the service provided at one of these centers. At King's College Hospital, the nurse counselor is present when the patient is told the diagnosis, this commonly being confirmed in the outpatient clinic by needle biopsy performed under local anesthesia. The patient often reacts to this information with shock, denial, and acute anxiety, and this inevitably leads to impaired concentration on the patient's part. For that reason, there is at this stage seldom more than the exchange of names and telephone numbers between the counselor and the patient, but nonetheless the patient may find that she derives comfort just from the nurse counselor's presence. The counselor then visits the patient at home before admission to hospital to make sure she understands the significance of the diagnosis and to help organize the practical aspects of her hospital stay. The woman may have to spend up to two weeks away from home, and this can in itself be a problem if she has young children. The interview is conducted according to the patient's needs and priorities, leaving it up to her to determine whether or not she yet wishes to explore her anxieties. Often, just the fact that the patient is given the opportunity to express fears and is encouraged to think in an objective manner about them seems to alleviate her distress. The dialogue between the patient and the counselor is continued on admission to the ward where the strange environment, coupled with fear about imminent surgery, often induces another increase in anxiety. At this stage, the patient needs to have practical information concerning preparation for surgery, and here the counselor's role is complementary to that of the ward staff. After the operation, counseling continues, and the various emotional stages through which the patient may progress are monitored. If the patient's reaction appears to be extreme, then specialist intervention is sought from a consultant psychiatrist who is a member of the team.

The counselor is usually standing by when the patient views her scar for the first time, since this is commonly reported to be a particularly stressful event within the postoperative period. The patient is given a temporary prosthesis before she is discharged from hospital, and arrangements are made for her to be provided with a permanent prosthesis six to eight weeks postoperatively. The selection of the most appropriate prosthesis is made by the patient herself, and the time at which this is introduced is determined by mutual agreement. If the prosthesis is introduced too early, some patients may react against it and reject it. Following discharge, a home visit is made two to three weeks later. By this time, any postoperative euphoria at having survived the operation should have evaporated, and the patient is beginning to come to terms with the reality of her experience in the quiet of her own home. When it is judged appropriate, regular contact between the patient and the counselor will cease. It is considered that the nurse counselor should be actively looking for the point at which she can withdraw, rather than perpetuating the contact and thus enforcing the idea that the patient is unable to cope independently (Denton & Baum, 1983).

In a short-term study of patients admitted for breast surgery, patients in one group were counseled preoperatively by a specialist nurse, while a control group received routine treatment. Anxiety levels were assessed preoperatively and then postoperatively in both groups (Cheeseman, Baum, & Ray, 1979). Counseled patients, whether they had benign or malignant disease, were found to be less anxious before the operation, although there were no differences apparent after surgery. The marked decline in anxiety by this stage for all groups suggested that the effects of counseling may here have been masked by postoperative euphoria. More relevant to a comprehensive evaluation of the specialist nurse's function, is Peter Maguire's study of long-term adjustment (Maguire, Tait, Brooke, Thomas, & Sellwood, 1980). Here, patients were assigned to either a control group receiving standard care or to a group who were given the support of a specialist nurse. The latter offered general counseling, monitored progress, and referred patients to a psychiatrist where indicated. Through monitoring, it was possible to detect most of those who needed psychiatric help, whereas such cases were generally undetected in the control group, and, as a result, psychiatric morbidity twelve to eighteen months postoperatively was significantly reduced. Patients were better adjusted, also, in terms of social recovery, return to work, adaptation to the loss of the breast, and satisfaction with their prosthesis (Maguire, Brooke, Tait, Thomas, & Sellwood, 1983). A similar evaluation of the service provided at King's College Hospital, described earlier, is currently under way, with psychological morbidity being assessed at one and two years postoperatively, and patients for whom counseling is provided being compared with others from whom it is withheld.

While the terms *specialist nurse* and *mastectomy counselor* are used interchangeably, it should be noted that the nurses do not generally receive formal, extensive training in counseling and therapeutic skills. They are qualified by their special experience to deal with a range of practical and emotional problems that mastectomy patients may have, but need to refer to a psychiatrist where there seems to be a significant difficulty in adjusting. In Maguire's study, the nurse's effectiveness in reducing morbidity indeed appeared to reside in her monitoring role and her alertness to the need of referral. Thus the specialist nurse does not, within current practice, provide the full support that is needed, and, to be effective, she must have the back-up of a psychological or psychiatric service.

Other Professionals

Professionals with training in psychology or social work can take a similar role to that of the specialist nurse. In one study of patients with cancer at three sites including the breast, information and support were provided by psychologists, social workers, and a psychiatric nurse over a period of six months, with referrals again being made where appropriate (Gordon et al., 1980). The intervention provided here was thus very much in line with the specialist nurse model. The counseled group showed a more rapid decline in anxiety, hostility, and depression; they were more active; and they were more realistic in their outlook, openly acknowledging the difficulties that they were facing because of their illness. Counseled patients thus seemed to show both reduced denial *and* less negative affect. The term *counseling* is a very broad one and can cover the range of aims and procedures, whoever is the provider. An alternative approach to intervention is to apply to the breast cancer setting structured therapeutic methods that have been evolved and tested for their efficiency in general psychological work. One advantage of this approach is that it defines the specific procedures being followed, and this means that these can then be more reliably applied by others if they are found to be effective.

An example of a structured intervention is that developed within Project Omega at Harvard Medical School. Newly diagnosed patients, with cancer at various sites including the breast, were randomly assigned to one of two treatment programs. Both of these focused on training patients to cope with the problems which faced them, encouraging strategies such as redefinition and confrontation which had been found to relate to low distress in previous research (see Chapter 3). In one intervention, patients were helped, first, to clarify the tasks or concerns that were of key importance to them; second, to generate strategies that might be employed to cope with these; and, third, to evaluate and rank the strategies generated for their practicability and the desirability of their consequences. Patients were, additionally, given some relaxation training. A second intervention also focused on handling concerns and tasks, but it was less structured and more explicitly encouraged patients to express their emotions. Both these interventions reduced distress, in comparison with a control group. Their effects were demonstrable at two, four, six, and even 12 months, in spite of the brevity of the interventions, with as few as four sessions being sufficient to alter adjustment significantly. In this study patients were screened using a questionnaire whose development is described in detail by Worden (1983), and those at high risk formed the main group for whom the interventions were provided. A selected group of low-risk patients were, however, also treated and these too were found to benefit. A package of tapes and a practitioner's manual describing the background research and the procedures adopted has been made available (Sobel & Worden, 1982).

Psychological interventions can also be useful in helping cancer patients to cope with particular aspects of the illness or its treatment. A general approach that could be employed in preparing patients for radiotherapy or chemotherapy is Stress Inoculation Training (SIT) (Meichenbaum & Jeremko, 1983), although no studies employing this have been reported to date. There is evidence, though, that more circumscribed techniques, such as systematic desensitization and relaxation training, can help reduce anticipatory nausea and vomiting and other adverse reactions to chemotherapy (Burish & Lyle, 1981; Morrow, 1981). It is unlikely that resources will be available to provide such interventions on a routine basis, but, with careful monitoring of patient's reactions at the beginning of treatment, it might be possible to offer them to patients who are most in need.

Rehabilitation Groups

These can deal not only with the physical and cosmetic aspects of the situation, but can help also to reconcile the patient to its emotional implications. Such groups are more common in the United States than in Great Britain. A format that is quite frequently adopted in the United States is that of the multidisciplinary team, perhaps comprising a nurse, a physical therapist or an occupational therapist, a social worker, and a Reach to Recovery volunteer (Letang, 1977; Schmid, Kiss, & Hibert, 1974; Winick & Robbins, 1977). Meetings are generally held while the patient is in hospital, with several meetings spanning the different kinds of problems that are relevant to the patient's situation. In these sessions, patients can be provided with information and can exchange ideas and also have the opportunity to see prostheses and to try out exercises. This feeling of active participation, and the comprehensiveness of the coverage that can be provided by such a group, is especially well received.

Hospital-based meetings provide an initial basis for adjustment, but many patients feel a need for some continued contact with a group beyond this time. Such groups may be led by a therapist, or can be self-help oriented, along the lines of the ostomy groups, and Halstead (1981) has described a self-help group for mastectomy patients. Whether led or not, such groups have a number of common benefits and hazards. One advantage is that they reinforce the knowledge that the person is not alone in having problems, and they allow her to see how others have experienced and dealt with these. Also, a key factor in the success of such groups is that each person not only has the role of someone who is helped but also the role of a helper. This can have its own therapeutic effect, and it has been found in other contexts that showing others how to cope with a problem often strengthens the person's own coping (Rakos & Schroeder, 1976). On the negative side, a possible risk is that people within the group who are strong deniers may find their defenses unacceptably challenged, and it has been suggested that "massive" deniers should perhaps be selected out from such groups (Speigel, 1979). Another risk is that there may be one or more people who keep bringing the discussion back to their personal anxieties, at best taking up a disproportionate amount of the group's time and, at worst, infecting the rest of the group with these. Group leaders should be aware of this as a potential problem and be armed with strategies for dealing with it. Finally, a common reservation about long-term groups concerns the possible effect of the group when one of its members suffers a recurrence or relapse, or dies. However, this is an argument against the existence of groups only where it is assumed that adjustment to the disease predicates an avoidance and denial of its implications. The fact of a continuing threat to health is one with which people are attempting to come to terms, and this should be a problem only where the group includes members who prefer not to acknowledge the threat. It is an argument, therefore, for the appropriate selection of patients entering such groups, rather than an argument against their existence. We have as yet little empirical information on the effectiveness of group support for breast cancer patients. Spiegel, Bloom, & Yalom (1981) have found that patients with metastatic disease, assigned randomly to a group, had lower mood disturbance and were more positive in their attitudes and coping than patients in a control group. Scher, Brick, Smalley, and Joseph (1977) observed that patients who regularly attended group therapy in a breast cancer clinic showed signs of psychological progress, but that many did not attend enough groups for significant change to occur. Much obviously depends on how the group is run and on the group members.

The Mastectomee as Helper

A potential source of support for the breast cancer patient can be other women who have gone through the same experience but who are now in good health and well adjusted to the mastectomy. A fellow mastectomee can empathize with the patient's immediate distress, reassure her in person that others have been through the same, and offer her hope for the future. The Mastectomy Association in the United Kingdom and the Reach to Recovery program, which began in the United States but is now to be found in several other countries, both provide volunteers who visit patients in hospital and at home and provide practical advice and emotional support. Many surgeons have expressed wariness about the possibility of some volunteers doing more harm than good, and it is important that there should be a screening process to make sure that those who are unsuitable are eliminated. If a volunteer has not adequately come to terms herself with the situation, she will be of little use to anyone else, and fear is contagious and can be easily transmitted to the new patient. A helper who has not resolved her own conflicts might also over-identify with the patient, seeing the latter's problems in terms of her own, and working through her own difficulties while imagining that she is helping the other (Kleiman, Mantell, & Alexander, 1977). It would be a pity, however, if such cautionary doubts were to result in all mastectomees being regarded as disqualified from a counseling role. Experimental studies of stress have shown that it is particularly valuable to have as a support someone who is going through the same experience. Schachter (1959) has argued that in such situations a key need is that of evaluating the status of our own feelings, and only another who is similarly placed can offer themselves as a suitable object of comparison. Also, if this person is calm and is coping effectively, then she can act as a model of what can be achieved, motivating the person under stress to emulate this response. Moreover, while there might be extra risks attached to counseling where the counselor is herself identified with the situation, it should be remembered that these risks are different only in degree rather than in kind from those that might be experienced by any helper, whether lay or professional. To resolve the controversy about the value of volunteer help, empirical studies are needed to evaluate critically the service provided and to establish, as in the case of formal counseling, that patients are indeed benefiting.

To summarize, routine medical and nursing care alone cannot meet the needs of patients who have to face the trauma of breast cancer and its treatment. Some patients fail to adjust, and these are often unnoticed, and thus are deprived of the psychiatric or psychological support that they require. Moreover, most patients experience problems to some degree, even if their general emotional state is not so badly affected that they would normally be referred for psychiatric help, and these people too may benefit from additional support. There are a number of ways in which this help has been provided. One way is through the services of a specialist nurse, working as part of the surgical team, who monitors patients' emotional state and liaises with a psychiatrist or psychologist to whom she makes referrals. Another is to screen patients to determine those at risk, and then to provide a psychological intervention aimed at stress management and/or training in cognitive and problem-solving skills. Finally, group therapy may be offered to all patients regardless of their reaction to the illness or their at-risk status. At present, it seems that the first two options are effective in reducing distress and promoting adjustment, while the effectiveness of group therapy, in the context of early breast cancer, and of volunteer support is still unclear. These approaches incorporate assumptions about who should be treated and when, and these are issues that need to be considered independently.

There are various criteria and strategies that can be considered when deciding *which* patients should be given such help.

1. Not all patients want additional support, and this was a claim made by the majority of patients in one survey (Downie, 1976). Those who refuse help may not be restricted to those who adjust well by themselves and without intervention. Worden and Weisman (1980) noted that refusers tended to be avoiders or deniers with respect to their illness, and the former strategy at least is one that is associated with poor adjustment (see Chapter 3). However, no patient can be pressured into taking part in a program, and *self-selection* is thus one criterion that must be taken into account.

2. Traditionally, only patients whose distress is noticed and judged to be of unusual degree are given special help. This *routine detection of need* misses many patients whose problems then remain unresolved.

3. Within the specialist nurse model, all patients can be provided with some support, and this alone might benefit patients if the nurse has the requisite counseling skills. Patients who fail to adjust are then referred for more intensive care, and it seems from the evidence to date that it is the nurse's capacity to *monitor all patients* and more reliably detect problems that reduces psychological morbidity.

4. An alternative would be to provide an *active intervention for all patients*, recognizing that all patients meet with some problems in adjusting, and that the process of adjustment can be facilitated even in patients who would cope reasonably well alone. A further advantage of this approach is its preventive nature. If a person has to wait until significant problems develop before intervention, maladaptive ways of coping may by then have become engrained and be difficult to modify. A disadvantage of the approach is its cost in terms of resources, and Worden (1983) has queried its cost effectiveness.

5. Finally, questionnaires or interviews can be used as soon as possible after diagnosis to predict patients at *high risk*, and support can be offered to these people only. This option is also preventive in nature, but it does assume that the greatest overall benefit is achieved by focusing resources upon those who

are the most disturbed. This group may not in practice be the only group who will respond, or even the group who will best respond, to the help offered. The woman who is moderately affected by her illness and mastectomy might benefit more than someone who is experiencing a variety of problems, or whose problems are extreme and deep seated. There is, indeed, some empirical evidence that interventions may be more effective in the case of patients who report fewer problems (Gordon et al., 1980). This is a question which needs further investigation.

The issue of *when* to counsel is in practice linked to the first issue of *whom* to counsel. With routine detection of need, or monitoring plus referral, problems will already have become established before help is provided, and there may be a resistance to change. In principle, a preventive orientation is preferable. Bard and Sutherland have claimed that discussion around the time of diagnosis can be of greater benefit than months of psychotherapy at a later date (1955) and, from the standpoint of crisis intervention theory also, early action is regarded as crucial. It is within the first few weeks that coping patterns are formed, and thus within this period that patients can best be influenced toward adaptive and away from maladaptive strategies (Caplan, 1974; Klein, 1971; Darbonne, 1967).

Social Support

The woman's own family and friends, in many circumstances, play a key role in helping her to adjust to her mastectomy and to her illness. The relationship that we have with others meets a number of our general psychological needs (Bloom, 1982a; Weiss, 1974). They provide a sense of identity, acceptance, and emotional security; they increase our feelings of self-worth and self-esteem; and, in time of stress, they can be a source of information, practical advice, and general emotional support. Studies of people's reactions to various kinds of crises have consistently shown that they are better able to withstand these where they have attachments with others, and an absence of this social support can make them more vulnerable to life stress at both physical and psychological levels (Caplan, 1981; Cobb, 1976; Dean & Lin, 1977). A number of writers have, however, pointed out that social contacts per se can be a mixed blessing in the context of illness (e.g., Dunkel-Schetter & Wortman, 1982). It is the quality rather than the availability of relationships with others that counts. Furthermore, even positive and apparently supportive behaviors can have a negative effect. The help and sympathy of others, no matter how well intended, can threaten autonomy, encourage dependency, and confirm the patient's view of herself as ill or damaged (Revenson, Wellman, & Felton, 1983; Satariano & Eckert, 1983; Suls, 1982). Nevertheless, one study of social support in the context of breast cancer found that perception of family cohesiveness and of social contact was positively related to adjustment, and seemed to discourage negative emotions and coping (Bloom, 1982b).

Many writers have pointed to the importance of a woman's relationship with her husband as a factor determining her adjustment to mastectomy (Cobliner,

1977; Ervin, 1973; Laxenaire, Bentz, & Chardot, 1972; Witkin, 1978), and a supportive husband can help women to cope with life stress in general. In a study of depression among women living in London, it was found that in many of the cases identified the person had faced a stressful life event in the previous nine months, for example, a threat to a relationship, an illness, or a major material loss (Brown & Harris, 1978). However, an important factor in determining whether or not such an event actually led to affective disorder was the presence or absence of a confiding relationship with a husband or boyfriend. With such a relationship, it seemed that women were less vulnerable and were protected against the psychological effects of loss or disappointment. It is important to note that it was the confiding nature of the relationship that was important and not just the existence of a husband or boyfriend, and marital status alone did not correlate with adjustment to breast cancer in Bloom's study (Bloom, 1982b).

Ideally, the woman with breast cancer can be helped to adjust by a partner who shares her experience, takes an active part in decisions, and encourages her to come to terms with what will, or has already, happened. He can also reassure her of his continued love and affection. One way of doing this is through humor. Such an attitude, against the background of a loving relationship, can serve better than any to minimize the significance of the loss of the breast.

> Patient: He didn't say a lot at first. He just looked at me and he said "Well, love, if it was for your body, I wouldn't have bothered marrying you." That's what he told me, he wouldn't have bothered, not a bit!

> Patient: He put his arm around me and he said "Never mind. Half a loaf is better than none." And I laughed and he laughed and, well, that did me more good than anything else. Honestly it did.

Indeed, too tender and over-protective an attitude might have a negative effect as suggested earlier, and in relation to breast cancer a specific area in which the husband may be too cautious is in his attitude to the scar. He may avoid confronting this both because of his own disquiet and because of his wife's modesty. As Renneker and Cutler (1953) point out, such a policy can reinforce the patient's "anxious concealment," and it may be better for both if an effort is made at an early stage to come to terms with the scar.

At the same time as recognizing the role that a husband can play in his wife's adjustment, his own possible concerns and conflicts must also be acknowledged. Many men suffer from psychosomatic symptoms during the pre and postoperative period (Pfefferbaum, Pashau, Jamison, & Wellisch, 1978; Wellisch et al., 1978), and husbands might benefit from some support at this time as well as their wives. They, too, may have difficulties in coming to terms with the disfigurement, and they, too, have to confront the fact of her cancer and the possibility that treatment might not, in the long term, prove successful. Several writers have suggested that sexual counseling should be provided for husbands and wives together (Wabrek & Wabrek, 1976; Wellisch et al., 1978; Witkin, 1978), and others have suggested that family members should be included in group work, meeting either with, or separately from, the patients themselves (Johnson &

Starr 1980; Spiegel, 1979; Gyllensköld, 1982). If the woman's family members have not come to terms with the illness, then they are unlikely to be able to help her to do so.

Summary

The nurse's role encompasses all aspects of patient care, but there are limits to the support she can offer. Patients may not look to the nurse for help with specific needs beyond their physical care and general reassurance, and they may mask their distress in order to play the role of good patient and to avoid overburdening staff. Furthermore, nurses as much as physicians feel the need to protect themselves emotionally by distancing themselves from patients' problems and their training does not at present equip them for a counseling role. One response to this situation has been to provide a specialist nurse who has a particular responsibility for psychological aspects of cancer care. Evidence suggests that this is effective in detecting and referring cases of psychological morbidity, where this would not otherwise be recognized. More recently, structured interventions have been employed by psychologists, to reduce stress and foster adaptive coping by training patients in relaxation and in cognitive skills that can be applied to the problems with which they are commonly confronted. These too reduce stress. Other alternative sources of support are groups or mastectomee volunteers; they can have drawbacks as well as advantages, and their general efficiency is yet to be determined. Aside from the nature of the intervention, other issues to be considered are the patients to whom it should most appropriately be offered, and the timing of the intervention. In general, a preventive orientation is to be preferred, rather than having to deal with established problems that may then be more difficult to modify.

Social support is important in any stressful situation, but it is the quality of the social relationships available that is important, and not just their availability per se. The husband's attitudes toward his wife's illness and mastectomy and the stability of the marital relationship are crucial in determining eventual adjustment. There is thus a case for involving husbands in any counseling that is offered, whether this is provided routinely or in response to a patient's failure to make a satisfactory psychological adjustment.

6

Cancer Attitudes and Related Behavior

Delay: A General Analysis

The psychological impact of breast cancer is important not only in considering women's reactions to diagnosis and treatment, but also their behavior when they discover a breast abnormality. A significant number of women delay seeking medical advice at this stage. Delay is usually defined as the interval that elapses from the time the symptom is first noticed to the time when the patient comes for a medical examination. It is often thought of in terms of discrete "blocks" of time, such as thirty days or less, one to three months, and three to six months. Many investigators have followed Pack and Gallo's example of arbitrarily defining an interval of more than three months as delay (Pack & Gallo, 1938), and at least 20 percent of women with breast symptoms wait for this or a longer time before consulting (Cameron & Hinton, 1968; Williams, Baum, & Hughes, 1976). Before looking at reasons for delay, it should be pointed out that there has been some controversy about its implications for effective treatment. Devitt (1976) has argued for a deterministic view of the disease's development, suggesting that there is little evidence that the interval between detection and treatment is an important variable in outcome. This viewpoint can, however, be challenged given that delay may itself depend upon the biological nature of the disease. A fast-growing cancer may alarm a woman by its sudden appearance and spur her into action, whereas a slower growing tumor may cause less alarm and be dealt with in a more leisurely fashion. Furthermore, the influence of delay on outcome may depend on the aggressiveness of the tumor: it may be of significance primarily in cancers of intermediate aggressiveness, where delay might allow the tumor to pass through that phase in its natural history when viable clonogenic cancer cells disseminate into the circulation. Disregarding the finer points of these discussions, the dissemination of cancer does occur over time, and it would seem reasonable to argue that even a cancer of low metastasizing potential may lead to death if diagnosis and treatment are excessively delayed. The value of prompt consultation has thus been an important theme in cancer education.

One approach to understanding delay is to relate this to illness behavior in general, and in this context it is important to make a clear distinction between illness and disease. Either can occur in the absence of the other (Herzlich, 1973; Idler, 1979). Disease is a concept referring to an objective physical or mental condition, pinpointed by objective signs. The condition may give rise to symptoms and these symptoms, by their characteristics, may help to identify the nature of the underlying disease, but they do not themselves define it. Illness, in contrast, is personally rather than scientifically defined and has a primarily subjective reality. It may or may not be related to an identifiable, objective dysfunction. An attribution of illness is made on the basis of the person's own experience of the state and of its implications for their present and future life, whereas a disease state is identified by analyzing the significance of signs and symptoms in the context of scientific, medical knowledge. The distinction between these two concepts is not just an academic one, but is important in understanding when and why people will seek medical care. They will do so only when they feel that they are *ill*, and this means that sometimes they will be seeking help in the absence of disease, and that at other times they will fail to do so in its presence.

What are the criteria people use in defining illness? Illness as a subjective state is quite closely related to *functional incapacity*. People may describe themselves as ill, and seek help, when they experience unpleasant symptoms, such as fatigue, nausea or pain, and the significance of such symptoms are increased where they affect social relationships, work or other activities (Zola, 1973). Herzlich argues that "the individual evaluates his condition not according to its intrinsic manifestations, but according to its effects" and "as long as one's activity is unhampered, physical phenomena are preceived but not thought of as illness, while the sense of being ill arises when everyday activity becomes difficult" (Herzlich, 1973, pp. 84, 80). Incapacity is not, however, the only criterion for determining illness. Any factor that leads to a suspicion of an underlying disorder plays a role. One such factor is *change*. Symptoms that have a recent onset are more likely to be defined as illness and to prompt consultation (Apple, 1960; Twaddle, 1969). The *ambiguity* of the symptom is also important. People are more likely to seek medical advice where the meaning of a symptom is unclear or if it has not been experienced previously (Apple, 1960; Banks & Keller, 1971). Factual beliefs about the hypothetical significance of symptoms in terms of disease have the effect of creating ambiguity and a desire for clarification.

There are wide differences among people in the number of consultations that they make over a given period. In one survey of 1400 patients in England and Wales (Cartwright, 1967), 25 percent were found to have been to their physician five or more times over a period of 12 months, while one-third had not consulted at all. Kessel and Shepherd (1965) studied 1500 patients in a London practice, and they similarly found a considerable variation. At one extreme, 3 percent of patients listed had not seen a physician for 10 years or more! Some of the variation may be due to differences in actual rates of illness, but this does not seem to be the full explanation. For example, those who usually do not see physicians have a more cautious attitude both in deciding whether they are going to be "ill" and whether a medical consultation is justified (Kessel & Shepherd, 1965). Differences among people are reflected not only in the ease with which they consult, or feel justification in consulting, but also in the nature of the criteria that they use in deciding whether or not to do so. Gordon (1966) concluded that people from lower socioeconomic groups are particularly likely to use functional incapacity as a criterion for "sick" status; and Zola's work has suggested similar kinds of differences on the basis of ethnic origin. In his studies, Americans of Irish descent or Anglo-Saxon descent were more likely to describe their problems in terms of specific physical dysfunction and interference with work, whereas, for Americans of Italian descent, the main complaints were diffuse feelings of pain and discomfort and interference with personal and social relations (Zola, 1973).

Some attempt to understand delay in the case of cancer can be made by referring to these kinds of factors. Functional incapacity is not an issue for most breast patients. They experience little in the way of pain or discomfort with their symptoms, and it does not interfere with everyday activity. Nor are the intrinsic features of the symptoms such as to cause concern. In many cases the lump may be gradual in onset, hardly noticeable at first and then slowly increasing in size. This means that a breast symptom is likely to give rise to concern only on the basis of a woman's beliefs about its possible implications. Without a factual knowledge that it might imply an underlying disease process, there would be little reason for her to give much thought to the symptom or to do anything about it. It is, then, primarily the suspicion of cancer that motivates and provides an incentive for consultation. However, in the case of a serious illness such as cancer, there is an additional factor not considered above that may greatly affect behavior. The decision to consult is made against the background of the fear evoked by cancer, and this fear can set up counter-forces that may prove to be stronger than its incentive effect. One way of conceptualizing this is to think of fear as eliciting two parallel response tendencies: danger control and fear control (Leventhal, 1970). The former refers to the adaptive coping strategies that the person brings to bear on the situation that poses the threat, in this context, prompt consultation to obtain an early diagnosis. Fear control, in contrast, refers to those ways of coping that center on the negative emotions brought by a recognition of threat, and which bypass the situation itself. Fear may be reduced by denying the danger, or putting it out of mind, and such a strategy would *discourage* consultation. Whether fear acts as an incentive or disincentive thus depends on the strategy the person adopts for coping with it.

Studies of Delay by Cancer Patients

With this general discussion of factors influencing illness behavior as background, we can now turn to specific studies of delay by cancer patients. A number of such studies have been carried out over the last three decades, and detailed reviews of this work have been presented (Blackwell, 1963; Green &

Roberts, 1974; Kutner, Makover, & Oppenheim, 1958). One commonly cited explanation for a failure to consult promptly is ignorance, in the form of either a lack of awareness of the possible implications of the symptom or of misconceptions such as a belief in the incurability of cancer or a belief that there is no cause to worry unless there is pain (Aitken-Swan & Paterson, 1955; Henderson, 1966; Cobb, Clark, McGuire, & Howe, 1954; Simmons & Daland, 1924). Somewhat paradoxically, there is also evidence of greater delay where cancer is suspected or where the person has had previous contact with a person with cancer (Cobb et al., 1954; Aitken-Swan & Paterson, 1955; Goldsen, 1963; Hacket, Cassem, & Raker, 1973), and many findings point directly to a fear of a diagnosis of malignancy or of treatment as a reason for delay (Aitken-Swan & Paterson, 1955; Gold, 1964; Henderson, 1966). Other factors that have been cited are modesty about the anticipated physical examination (Gold, 1964; Henderson, 1966); an unsatisfactory relationship with the physician; and domestic reasons, such as holidays, family weddings or being unable to leave the house (Aitken-Swan & Paterson, 1955; Bacon, Renneker, & Cutler, 1953; Henderson, 1966). There are some demographic differences between delayers and nondelayers: the former are more likely to have a low-income and socioeconomic status, and a poor education (Goldsen, 1963; Hacket et al., 1973; Kutner & Gordan, 1958).

These studies have dealt with patients who have cancer in various sites, but it is likely that the factors responsible for delay differ depending on the nature of the symptom, its functional implications, the level of general knowledge about its possible signifiance, and expectations of treatment and control were cancer to be diagnosed. For this reason, a number of studies have focused exclusively on responses to symptoms in a particular site or have separated patients according to the type of cancer. The methods and findings of such studies of delay in *breast* cancer patients are summarized in Table 6.1.

There would seem to be three principal reasons for these patients' delay, which together summarize and account for the findings. The first is a *lack of awareness* of the implications of the breast symptom and the importance of early treatment. Even in the 1950s it could be stated that "every adult woman knows what a *lump* in the breast *may* mean. Ignorance is rare . . . ." (Paterson, 1955, p. 934); yet delayers, according to their self-reports, are less likely to have thought of the possibility of cancer or to have seen the symptom as a cause for concern (Cameron & Hinton, 1968; Eardley, 1974; Williams et al., 1976). Delayers tend to be of lower social class and education levels and to be from older age groups (Cameron & Hinton, 1968; Greer, 1974; Williams et al., 1976), and this offers some support for an explanation in terms of ignorance, since surveys have shown that these are the groups that are most likely to be uninformed or misinformed about cancer (Briggs & Wakefield, 1966; Knopf, 1974). The second reason for delay is *unconscious denial* of the implications of the breast symptom and of the need to seek medical advice. Interviews with cancer patients often show a denial and avoidance of an awareness of cancer, or denial and suppression of the emotions that would normally be associated with it. This kind of response is positively related to delay, while defenses such as intellectualization and isolation are, in contrast, negatively related (Margarey et al., 1977; Worden & Weisman, 1975).

Table 6-1. Reasons for Delay and Characteristics of Delayers in Patients with Breast Abnormalities

Sugar and Watkins, 1961	Delayers showed little fear or knowledge of cancer; also depression and indifference. Anxiety resulted in prompt consultation.
Gold, 1964	Delay was associated with ignorance regarding cancer, absence of pain, fear of cancer, and a hope that the lump would go away.
Hammerschlag, 1964	Delayers had well-defined "body boundaries."
Cameron and Hinton, 1968	Delayers felt little or no anxiety about the tumor, gave fear and domestic reasons for delay, were more introverted, and had less education.
Eardley, 1974	Delayers were less likely to have thought of cancer on discovery of the symptom and were less likely to mention the advantage of early consultation. Knowledge and concern about the possible seriousness of the lump, fear of cancer, discomfort, the influence of others, and chance factors acted as triggers for action.
Greer, 1974	Delayers saw their symptoms as less serious. They were fearful of cancer and had a fatalistic attitude toward its outcome. They were fearful of treatment, and of losing the breast, and were deniers of life crises.
Williams et al., 1976	Delayers were characterized by absence of pain and ignorance of the possible severity of the condition. They feared the diagnosis of cancer and its consequences. Age, parity, and educational attainment were also factors.
Worden and Weisman, 1975[a,b]	Delayers tended to avoid the term *cancer*, and showed high manifest anxiety, tension, fatigue, and confusion, and high vulnerability.
Margarey et al., 1977	Delayers showed more denial, suppression, depression and nonverbal anxiety, and less conscious anxiety and intellectualization—isolation
MacArthur and Smith, 1981[b]	Delayers' symptoms were more likely to be ambiguous.

[a] This study included also patients with cancer at other sites, but the data for the breast group were separately analyzed.

[b] Patients with malignant disease only. All studies included patients with both benign and malignant disease, except for those so marked.

It seems that delayers are, moreover, predisposed to denial as a way of coping with threat, and have habitually employed this in past situations (Greer, 1974). It should be noted, though, that Hammerschlag, Fisher, DeCosse, & Kaplan (1964) failed to find a relationship between delay and repression scores on the Minnesota Multiphasic Personality Inventory (MMPI). The third principal reason for delay is a *conscious fear and avoidance* of the diagnosis of cancer and of its implications. Although some investigators have concluded that conscious fears play a minor role only (Cameron & Hinton, 1968; Margarey et al., 1977), others have attributed delay to fear of mastectomy (Gold, 1964; Greer, 1974); fear of malignancy (Buls, Jones, Bennett, & Chan, 1976; Gold, 1964; Greer, 1974; Williams et al., 1976); and to a general fear of hospitalization or surgery (Gold, 1964). Delayers have also been found to have higher scores on a planning and organizational dimension of personality, reflecting a disposition to behave in a considered rather than an impulsive fashion (Ray & Baum, 1979), and other findings suggest that they are independent, self-steering and goal-oriented (Fisher, 1967; Hammerschlag et al., 1964). People with these characteristics would be expected to be more vulnerable to the inhibiting effect of fear since, as Eardley (1974) has noted, many of those women who consult promptly do so automatically, without considering what the implications of either consultation or a failure to consult might be. Finally, while a lack of awareness, unconscious denial and conscious fear and avoidance may be the most common factors in delay, there may be other factors that are of overriding importance in individual cases. They would include a reluctance to be examined (Greer, 1974; Williams et al., 1976) and domestic difficulties or commitments (Cameron & Hinton, 1968; Greer, 1974).

These conclusions seem well supported, but it is worth noting that the general area is one that is fraught with methodological difficulties. To begin with, all patients must be interviewed retrospectively. The focus of interest is their feelings and appraisals before consultation, but their experiences since so doing will add new information (Chesser & Anderson, 1975) and thus influence the assessment. Other sources of contamination could differentially affect delayers and nondelayers. One is the possibility that people's self-reports are biased to make them acceptable both socially and personally. Delay has negative connotations, in implying that the patient's behavior has somehow been blameworthy. It has indeed been suggested that the more neutral word "lagtime" should be used instead of delay, in order to avoid these value implications (Worden & Weisman, 1975). Patients who have delayed may, additionally, fear that they have made matters worse, and be self-reproachful. Through embarrassment and guilt, therefore, they may rationalize their behavior, for example, by claiming ignorance, and so justifying their delay to themselves and to the interviewer. Another common type of observation, that delayers at the time of interview are more anxious (Cameron & Hinton, 1968), helpless and hopeless (Sugar & Watkins, 1961), or depressed, angry, confused and fatigued (Margarey et al., 1977), might also be challenged on similar grounds. These characteristics are interpreted as factors that *cause* delay, but they could equally well be regarded as the outcome of the person's awareness that she might have behaved more wisely. An alternative approach to investigations of delay, which avoids arousing feelings of guilt or embarrassment and therefore runs less risk of biasing patients' reports and demeanor, is to look for "triggers to action" rather than reasons for delay. This follows a lead provided by Zola (1973) in the field of general illness behavior and by Eardley (1974) in the context of cancer delay. This kind of approach has the added benefit that it makes it evident that factors that are proffered as explanations for delay, most obviously a fear of cancer, can also be a reason for prompt consultation (Cameron & Hinton, 1968; Eardley & Wakefield, 1976; Henderson, 1966).

The three main explanations of delay in breast cancer patients, suggested above, are supported by different kinds of evidence, and this makes them fairly robust in spite of these problems of interpretation. They also have a certain face validity, in that they plausibly suggest corresponding portraits of typical delayers. The first would be that of a woman who is from a lower social class, has received little formal education, and is in her forties or over. She is poorly informed about cancer and about health issues in general. This woman would be most likely to ask about her breast lump when visiting her physician for some other reason, or at a stage when it is causing some discomfort. Being unaware of the symptom's possible significance she might be little distressed at the stage of presentation, and be quite surprised when it is evidently regarded as being of some significance by the general practitioner. The second type would be exemplified by the woman who is relatively well informed about health issues including cancer, but does not spend time dwelling on them. She might have an abstract knowledge, but does not think of herself in relation to these facts. Cancer for her is a dreadful disease, but not one that causes actual fear since she has not really considered herself as a potential victim. When she discovers a breast symptom she may intellectually recognize the association between this and cancer, but not seriously consider it as a possibility in her own case. If she has had benign lumps before, then she may convince herself that this, too, is benign; or she may rationalize that all women develop lumps from time to time and that they are not worth worrying about unless they show signs of development. She may successfully put the symptom out of mind, or put off going to the physician "for the time being." Finally, some trigger counters these defenses and directs her toward the physician. Her husband may keep reminding her about the lump and press her to go, or she may read a magazine article that clearly describes her situation and prevents further self-deception. The third type would be represented by a woman who is similarly well educated and well informed about health issues. She does take these personally and may conscientiously follow a number of preventive recommendations such as watching her diet or her smoking. She is used to making her own decisions and does not respond unthinkingly to external pressures. If she discovers a breast symptom her first reaction is one of alarm at its implications. If she is aware that the majority of breast lumps are, in fact, benign, she may consult immediately in order to reassure herself. If, however, she fears that a consultation may confirm and make immediate that which she now dreads, she may procrastinate. She recognizes that she ought to seek advice, but finds it difficult to bring herself to do so. She may openly acknowledge her fear and reluctance. On the other hand, she may protect her self-image by constructing "good" reasons for her delay, reassuring herself that she will go to the physician just as soon as holidays, family occasions, or work pressures, etc., permit. These descriptions, of course, are of ideal types, and in practice any individual case of delay may comprise a combination of ignorance, denial, and conscious fear and avoidance.

The Value of Breast Self-Examination and Screening

Efforts to foster early diagnosis and treatment have comprised not only appeals to women to consult promptly when they discover a breast abnormality; they are also aimed at the earlier *detection* of symptoms. Two approaches are possible here: the first is to screen an asymptomatic, at-risk population, and the second, to educate women to examine themselves systematically and to report any abnormal findings promptly. Both approaches have attracted professionals and politicians alike, so much so that many have accepted their value as an article of faith, yet they should be subjected to scientific scrutiny in the same way as any other clinical intervention, to determine whether they do actually result in a reduction in deaths.

Screening

For the lay person, it may seem inconceivable that screening can do anything but good, yet possible disadvantages must be considered and weighed against possible benefits. First, a negative finding on a first examination could lead to a false sense of security, and women who feel this might then be at greater risk of delay if they are not invited back at regular intervals for follow-up examinations or if they decline such invitations. Second, screening programs generate an increased biopsy rate, since many women with lumpy breasts due to benign disorders are referred to the surgeon for operative procedures. Even the smallest breast operation causes psychological stress and, as with a very large number of any type of operation, there might be a percentage of surgical and anesthetic mishaps. Also, we have to consider the risk of low doses of ionizing radiation affecting the breast. There is no agreed safe dose of radiation, so it must be recognized that there is a very small risk of inducing cancers by submitting women to repeated mammograms at regular intervals, extending over a period of perhaps 30 years. These risks have probably been exaggerated, and, with new techniques that deliver a very low dose of radiation for a complete set of mammograms, most experts feel that the risk has been reduced to a safe minimum. Another nagging anxiety about screening programs is the number of abnormalities of marginal significance now being detected. The pathological diagnosis is not always clear, and many small lesions detected by mammography alone on biopsy demonstrate minimal changes on the borderline between epithelial overgrowth, intraduct cancer, and invasive cancer. For all we know, the screening program may be "causing" cancer by the diagnosis of latent disease which, if left alone, would never express the invasive potential of a clinically apparent breast cancer. Often the pathologist and the surgeon are in doubt as to what should be the definitive management of such cases, and it is likely, therefore, that in any large-scale screening program a number of mastectomies will be carried out because of these abnormalities. This could, in theory, increase the mastectomy rate within the population without influencing the mortality rates from breast cancer.

Furthermore, there are two artifacts that make the interpretation of the results from screening programs difficult. The first of these artifacts is referred to as *lead time*. This is the interval between the diagnosis at screening and the diagnosis when clinical signs are apparent to the patient, and it has been estimated that this may vary anything between six months and six years. Intervention earlier in the natural history of the disease inevitably prolongs the period of observation, even if the treatment has not influenced the outcome. The survival after mastectomy in such cases would be prolonged (case fatality rates) without necessarily influencing the mortality rates for the whole population. The second artifact is known as *length bias*. For simplicity's sake, assuming that there are two types of breast cancer, a fast-growing and a slow-growing variety, the fast-growing and more lethal form of the disease is likely to present itself between screening intervals, whereas the slow-growing disease with the better prognosis is likely to be detected at screening intervals. Therefore, cancers detected at screening are likely to be biologically favorable with, again, an improved survival following local treatment.

For these reasons, the only possible way of evaluating the impact of a screening program is to conduct a randomized trial between matched screened and nonscreened populations, using the mortality rates for breast cancer over the period of observation as the index of success. The first of such studies was established by the Health Insurance Plan in New York just over 10 years ago (Shapiro, Venet, Strax, Venet, & Roesse, 1982). Women subscribing to this plan were divided randomly into two groups, 31,000 in each. One group received annual screening by mammography and clinical examination, and the other group was used as a control population and allowed to come forward with their breast cancers by self-detection. As might have been predicted, smaller cancers with a lower incidence of involvement of lymph nodes were picked up among the screened population, with an ultimately significant but small reduction in the mortality rate from breast cancer among this group. Unfortunately, the benefit seemed only to apply to women over the age of 50. Even among the screened population, cancers that appeared to be of the more aggressive type developed between the fixed screening intervals, reducing though by no means abolishing the benefits of the annual screen that was demonstrated by the whole of the test population. With the improvements in mammographic techniques over the last ten years, and the difficulty in calculating the cost effectiveness of such a strategy on a nationwide basis, it has become imperative to repeat this experiment. Currently, a number of such studies are underway in Canada and in Sweden. As a result of the ethical dilemma with such programs, it has been impossible to repeat this study systematically in the United States, and various uncontrolled evaluations are being conducted there. In the United Kingdom, a compromise solution has been adopted, and the Department of Health and Social Security (DHSS) is currently funding a study comparing regular screening with public health education and self-examination, using defined geographical areas for the control and test populations (UK Trial of Early Detection of Cancer Group, 1981).

Breast Self-Examination

In theory at least, breast self-examination (BSE) might be a more fruitful and a less costly exercise than screening by mammography. The growth patterns of solid tumors can be described by a complex Gompertzian function (a pattern of growth that starts off as an exponential function, but ends with a plateau). Screening by mammography might detect cancers with a minimum diameter of, say, 0.25 cm, that is two doublings before the smallest lump detectable by palpation alone. Breast self-examination might detect all lumps between 1 and 4 cm (that is the next two doublings), which still remain at an operable stage. If the doubling time increases with the size of the primary tumor, as might be expected in the later component of a Gompertzian growth curve, then the time available for dissemination is in theory greater for the period covered by breast self-examination than that for mammographic screening. In the experience of most clinicians in the United Kingdom, about 25 percent of women with breast cancer have inoperable tumors, 5 cm or more in maximum diameter. So, perhaps before we invest huge resources into screening the whole female population to detect cancers less than 1 cm in diameter, we might turn our attention to persuading women to present themselves with tumors between 1 and 4 cm diameter. This subject has been more fully dealt with in a recent critical review (Baum, 1982). As already stated, the UK DHSS is currently funding a trial to determine whether breast self-examination can save lives, but it will be many years before any definitive data are available.

Changing Attitudes and Behavior

Behavioral Outcomes of Programs for BSE and Screening

It was not until the 1970s that health educators began systematically to assess the impact of education on behavior. There is now evidence that teaching programs on BSE can influence opinions on the advantages of early treatment and on the possibility of early detection, but with disappointing little change in the extent to which BSE is adopted (Hobbs, Haran, Pendleton, Jones, & Posner, 1984). As part of the DHSS study previously mentioned (Calnan, Chamberlain, & Moss, 1983; Calnan, 1984a), it was found that classes had an effect on technique and confidence rather than frequency of practice. Factors affecting attendance also were studied. Those who attended classes following invitation were more likely than nonattenders to see themselves as vulnerable to breast cancer, and to admit to concern, and a history of other preventive behaviors and use of preventive services was another good predictor. The same factors were related to acceptance of an invitation for breast screening in a separate sample of women. In a survey connected with this study many women cited a preference for screening over breast self-examination (Calnan, 1984b). They felt that screening would be more reliable, being carried out by specialized staff, and were also deterred by the prospect of public classes in BSE and the embarrassment that they associated with these. It is also interesting that 43 percent of those surveyed held a rather negative stereotype of the breast self-examiner, seeing her typically as neurotic, hypochondriacal, frightened, and a worrier.

People vary in their health-related behavior and in their responsiveness to education programs. In broad, sociodemographic terms, a number of studies suggest that women take preventive action more readily than men, especially where this requires medical intervention (Nathanson, 1977), and groups with higher levels of education, income and socioeconomic status are more prevention-oriented than others (Fink, Shapiro, & Lewison, 1968; Haefner, Kegeles, Kirscht, & Rosenstock, 1967). This may be in part because services and information are more accessible to these groups, and class differences are reduced if facilities are made more easily available (Hobbs, 1980). Another influence is attitudes related to health care. For example, Antonovsky and Anson (1976) interviewed attenders at a breast clinic and a group of controls, and divided them on the basis of the interviews into four categories: conformists—who were unconditionally trusting and dependent on authority figures and responded to external pressures; the rational goal-oriented type—who had an instrumental attitude toward physicians and health care services and would respond to an invitation to attend the clinic if persuaded it was worthwhile; the complaisant stoic—who, while she had a generally positive attitude toward health care, had no personal investment in this and would only attend if she had a clear symptom or some other personal incentive; and those who the researchers described as ambivalent-anxious—who combine high levels of anxiety with a shifting attitude toward physicians and health care. Regular attenders at the breast clinic were more likely to come from the first and second categories. Women in the last group tended to be afraid of examinations or thought that they were pointless as a means of reducing the threat of cancer and were least likely to attend regularly.

A number of authors have raised the question of whether health education might have negative psychological effects, producing undue anxiety or cancerophobia. General practitioners contacted in one early survey (Wakefield & Davidson, 1958) were in favor of direct talks to the public and formal education programs. They regarded this approach as preferable to general media coverage of such issues, and none felt the overall effects to be harmful. Psychiatrists' opinions were sought in another study (Horn, 1956), and few of these took the view that education increases anxiety or that such anxiety would result in more harm than good. Many writers associated with cancer education have similarly claimed that adverse effects are not a problem. Such opinions are, however, no more than opinions; they are founded on unsystematic observation and their validity could well be challenged by empirical research. The fact that a greater awareness of the threat of cancer causes anxiety in *some* people is undeniable. What is in question is the extent of such an effect in the context of health education, and the significance of the effect in relation to the advantages of an increased awareness. The World Health Organization (1964) has defined health as "a state of complete physical, mental and social well being," and any evaluation of health education programs should monitor their psychosocial as well as physical outcomes.

Maximizing Change

To persuade someone to follow a course of action, there are a number of factors that need to be considered. A message that is presented with this aim is effective only if (1) it is assimilated, (2) it is credible, (3) it motivates compliance, and (4) the motivation to comply can be translated into action.

Assimilation

The first objective is that the message should be heard and retained. It must be attention-worthy since, if it is not registered in the first place, it is unlikely to be recalled subsequently. It must also be comprehensible. The difficulties that lay people have with some medical terms have already been described, and these and all but the simplest vocabulary should be avoided. Another consideration often neglected is sentence structure. Many messages presented to the public are so complex that they are beyond the capacities of all but a few. Thus any appeal for self-examination or screening must ensure that the women to whom it is directed feel that it is of relevance to them, and ensure also that it is within their comprehension.

Credibility

Social psychologists in the 1950s and 1960s explored in depth those characteristics of the source and the message that facilitate attitude change (e.g., Hovland, Janis, & Kelly, 1953). Key factors are the communicator's perceived authority and trustworthiness. There can be no room for doubt about the latter's expertise nor about the integrity of the motives that lie behind the attempt to persuade. It is unlikely that the motives of a communicator would, in fact, be in question in the context of health education compared, say, with advertising or politics, but a lack of conviction can be a problem where the audience is aware of, or believes there to be, an absence of consensus within the scientific community on the themes dealt with by the message. This could be an issue for cancer education, were the public to become aware of controversy about the value of screening and self-examination, and hence the need for the evaluation studies in progress. Researchers have also debated the relative effectiveness of different ways of presenting the message itself, whether it should present its own counter-arguments and in return refute these (for example, "some people believe that cancer is incurable") or whether it should ignore alternative viewpoints. It seems that there is no simple answer to this, and that the optimal form of presentation varies, depending on the degree and nature of resistance anticipated and the sophistication of the audience. Thus, as Rosenstock (1960) and others have argued, it is important that the content of any program should take into account the prevailing attitudes of the population to whom it is directed. Unfortunately, this population is not homogenous, and then the primary targets within the population have to be identified. An approach that sways one section may fail to influence another and vice versa.

Motivating Compliance

Attitude change in itself does not always result in a change in behavior, and social psychologists have for many years been aware that the correlation between these two sets of variables is in some cases low (Wicker, 1969). One reason for this is that any single action is multidetermined. Behavior is influenced by the full range of beliefs the person holds about an action's perceived consequences, and the way in which these are evaluated, and not by any single attitude in isolation (Fishbein & Ajzen, 1980). It is influenced also by the norms or standards of the group to which the person belongs and by the latter's motivation to comply with social pressures and constraints. As a result, an appeal may be persuasive in the sense of convincing the person of the validity of the message, yet still not result in compliance because of the existence of competing attitudes and inhibitions.

As already indicated, if a message is to be attended to in the first place, it cannot deal solely with the transmission of knowledge in the abstract, but must indicate clearly that the risk is real and relevant to that person. As a result, it focuses attention on a threat of whose existence the person may have been unaware or which they have been choosing to ignore. The role of threat in communication and persuasion is a complex one. It can be both an incentive and a disincentive for compliance, just as fear can encourage or discourage consultation in the context of delay (see p. 71). Its effect has been widely explored within the laboratory. Experimental studies have included attempts to persuade people to stop smoking (Leventhal & Watts, 1966); to have tetanus injections (Leventhal, Singer, & Jones, 1965); to take care of their teeth and gums (Janis & Feshbach, 1953); to wear seat belts (Berkowitz & Cottingham, 1960); and to drive safely (Rogers & Mewborn, 1976). The experimental design in these studies typically involves a manipulation of the degree of threat implicit in the message, and the findings have shown that increases in threat can *either* facilitate or inhibit changes in attitudes and behavior. Leventhal's differentiation between danger and fear control was introduced when we were discussing delay, and it is relevant here also. An appeal that points to a danger is likely to elicit fear, and its effectiveness depends on whether the recipient is motivated primarily to control the danger or to control the fear associated with this. If the fear elicited is sufficiently great, then fear control may be the dominant tendency and instrumental coping (danger control) may be ignored, thus neutralizing any movement toward a change in attitudes or behavior. Fear appeals in these circumstances can even have a "boomerang" effect, if they result in someone paying even less attention to the threat than they would previously have done, because it is now too upsetting to take the danger seriously or to contemplate it as relevant to their own situation. In practice, one way to motivate danger control while at the same time countering fear is to emphasize the benefits of following the recommendation rather than the negative consequences of not doing so. Thus, Kirscht, Haefner and Ereland (1975), in an attempt to persuade people to attend for a general health screening, found that a message that emphasized how easy it was to get checked, and the benefits of this in terms of a better chance of continued good health, was more effective than a relatively threatening message that emphasized the possibility of being sick without knowing it and the negative aspects of sickness. Many cancer education programs also implicitly recognize the value of this kind of positive approach (Hart, 1972; Hobbs, 1980) and focus on the role of the recommended action in averting threat by offering a firm hope of cure should a malignancy be detected at an early stage. In the specific case of breast cancer, the communication can also make clear that, while any changes in the breast should be investigated as early as possible, these usually prove to be benign rather than malignant.

The goal of such messages is to reconcile the two aims of raising an alarm, without which there is no incentive for change, and offering reassurance, without which there may be every incentive for ignoring the message in order to restore peace of mind.

Translation into Action

The final objective to be met in health education is to ensure that the motivation to comply, once engendered, results in action. Often, an inclination to behave in a certain way is never fulfilled, because of inertia or because of obstacles that make it difficult to put the inclination into practice. This constitutes yet a further reason for the low correlation observed between attitudes and behavior referred to earlier. To cross what Baric has referred to as the *action threshold* (1979), a health appeal must provide a specific plan of action that can be put into practice, rather than merely identifying aims, and any barriers to the plan's possible implementation must be removed. Thus, there is little point in convincing women of the benefits of screening if the facilities themselves are not easily obtainable, nor of motivating them to examine their breasts if they are uncertain how to go about this. In situations where no clear course of action is recommended or where it cannot be put into practice, control of the danger portrayed is not possible, and the woman is more likely to resort instead to fear control: the message will then produce denial or avoidance rather than behavior change.

A General Model

Strictly speaking, consultation after discovery of a breast abnormality is an illness behavior, that is, "any activity undertaken by a person who feels ill, to define the state of his health and to discover a suitable remedy" (Kasl & Cobb, 1966, p. 246), while screening and breast self-examination are *health* behaviors, in the sense that they are undertaken in the absence of illness although not necessarily in the absence of disease (see p. 70). This distinction between symptomatic and asymptomatic behaviors, however, may have little significance when it comes to understanding the factors that influence them; for example, perception of risk and fear are two factors that we have had to consider in both contexts. It may then be possible to look at all these behaviors within a common framework. One of the most fruitful analyses in this area has been the Health Belief Model, originally proposed by Rosenstock (1966). It has most often been applied in situations where there are no symptoms, since it was initially oriented toward the theme of prevention (and has even provided a conceptual framework for an understanding of family planning behavior: Katatsky, 1977). In practice, however, it is applicable also to situations that involve actual illness, and the model has been used to analyze responses both to early symptoms and to chronic illness (Becker, 1974; Becker & Maiman, 1975; Kasl, 1974; Leavitt, 1979). It offers a conceptual framework for organizing the many and diverse variables that have been involved in the explanation of health and illness behavior, and it has received some empirical support, although this is sufficiently inconsistent to raise queries about either the completeness of the model or the way it has been applied.

There are four principal factors detailed within the model. The first relates to the person's perception of his or her own vulnerability to the illness, sometimes interpreted as the subjective probability of its occurrence. The second is the perceived severity of the illness. These two factors together determine the degree of personal risk or threat experienced. The third factor concerns perceived benefits of the action that is recommended in order to avert the threat, while the fourth considers the action's feasibility in terms of relevant disincentives and barriers. The latter could be financial or practical difficulties, or less tangible costs such as physical discomfort, anxiety, social disapproval, or embarrassment. Taken together, the third and fourth factors determine readiness to take the particular action recommended, depending upon the balance between the benefits and the costs it promises. A further factor that has been noted, but that usually receives less attention than the others, is the need for some stimulus that prompts the translation of a readiness to take an action into actual behavior. This could be an internal trigger or an external cue such as pressure from other people.

One common criticism of the Health Belief Model is its neglect of emotions as factors in health and illness behaviors. Perceptions and expectations alone are cast as the motivators, yet as has been emphasized throughout this chapter, fear can act together with these factors to reinforce action in some circumstances and inhibit it in others. Moreover, the concept of fear control introduces a dynamic element into the system, since fear can act to modify initial perceptions and expectations. A perception of threat may lead to fear which, if it cannot be tackled by coping focused on the danger itself, may be defended against by reassessing the threat. In this way perceptions may be brought into line with a policy of nonaction, and this is an alternative outcome to be considered alongside that of behavior being changed to correspond with the perception of threat. The Health Belief Model, as it stands, is a static one, and does not allow for such dynamic adjustments in perceptions. With this revision it can, however, provide a conceptual framework for the analysis both of behaviors such as attendance at screening clinics and breast self-examination, and of delay:

1. Perceived vulnerability: only the woman who sees herself as personally at risk from breast cancer is likely to take measures aimed at early detection, and only the woman who recognizes the potential significance of a breast symptom will be motivated to consult promptly about this.
2. Perceived seriousness of the illness: this is possibly a fairly constant factor in the case of cancer, given the general stereotype, and there would be few women who would not regard the disease as constituting a grave threat.
3. Perceived benefits of action: here there is greater variability. Within the population as a whole there is evidence of some optimism about curability given early detection and diagnosis, but there are many people who are more pessimistic. The woman who believes that treatment is generally ineffective has little incentive to take action, whether for early detection or diagnosis, regardless of the degree of threat perceived.

4. Perceived disincentives and barriers: practical considerations may deter women from attending screening clinics and surgeries, and doubts about ability to self-examine would provide an obvious disincentive to practice this. Emotional costs are, however, likely to be more significant, particularly in the case of delay. Here there is a distinct possibility that the woman's fears will be confirmed, and the "cost" of a diagnosis of cancer and the treatment that would follow may outweigh the perceived benefits of action. Even for the woman who is symptom-free, screening or self-examination may cause embarrassment or elicit anxieties that will deter her from this action.

5. The effect of fear: if the costs outweigh the benefits for the person concerned, and action is inhibited, an acknowledgment of the threat would engender its own anxiety. To resolve this, the woman may reappraise the threat consciously or unconsciously and devalue her personal risk.

Summary

The woman who delays does so against a background of either ignorance or fear. In some cases there may be a genuine failure to recognize the possible significance of the symptom. In others, the fear prompted by too acute an awareness of danger can itself inhibit action. The woman may be motivated to try to reduce this fear, rather than to resolve the danger itself, by unconsciously denying the possibility of cancer or consciously avoiding consulting and the chance of having her suspicions confirmed.

Programs for breast screening and self-examination have also to counter both ignorance and fear. To motivate action, any message must make explicit the fact that every woman is at risk. This can, however, cause alarm, and the response to this may be to put the message out of mind or to discount its import.

The Health Belief Model provides a framework for understanding both preventive and symptomatic behavior. Within the model, the incentive to action is provided by the degree of threat perceived, which is in turn dependent on the perceived seriousness of the illness and the person's beliefs about personal vulnerability. However, action is not actually taken if it is seen as ineffective in averting threat or where the practical and emotional costs are too high. To change attitudes and behavior, therefore, it is important not just to emphasize the threat of cancer, but also to reduce disincentives by emphasizing the benefits of early detection and diagnosis and allaying the alarm that most women feel in thinking of themselves as potential victims. Unfortunately, this last objective may be difficult to achieve with integrity, while the prospect of effective treatment is uncertain and while the treatments available are in themselves toxic or mutilating.

7

Cancer: A Psychosomatic Disease?

Psychological factors can affect illness outcome through their influence on behavior when a symptom is discovered, and their influence on behaviors aimed at early detection. Can they, in addition, play a role in the etiology of the disease itself? The ability of the psyche to affect the body and its processes is widely recognized, and the concept of psychosomatic illness reflects this recognition. However, traditionally, the label *psychosomatic* is applied to a limited number of illnesses, such as peptic ulcers and heart disease, and this implies that there exists a category distinct from these to which the label does not apply and in whose case these influences are absent. Such a view is no longer acceptable, and in current theories and research it is assumed that psychological factors play a role in a variety of illness contexts.

Stress and General Illness Susceptibility

There have been many attempts to portray the personality characteristics of the "typical" sufferer from various diseases. These portraits have in some cases gained wide public acceptance, but the concept of a relationship between highly specific psychological characteristics of the person and particular diseases does not always meet with empirical support, and the role of personality is, on the whole, today less emphasized in theory and research. One exception is the case of the "coronary prone personality" (Byrne, 1978; Friedman, 1969; Glass, 1977), and there is now increasing acceptance of a "cancer prone personality," of which more will be said later. Recent interest has tended, in general, to shift away from factors defined primarily with the individual and has turned toward the effects of external influences in the form of life events and changes. This shift in emphasis has been facilitated, and encouraged, by the development of an appropriate questionnaire, the "Schedule of Recent Experience" (Holmes & Rahe, 1967). This comprises a list of life events, ranging from death of a spouse or divorce at one extreme to minor violations of the law at the other, and the subject is required to check those events that he or she has recently experienced. Both desirable and undesirable events are included in this list, since it is the fact of having to accommodate to change rather than wider, evaluative implications of the event that were regarded by the authors as most significant in the etiology of illness. In the published questionnaire, each event has associated with it an estimate of the amount of readjustment that it would require. These estimates were obtained from a group of judges who were asked to give values for each event, on the basis that "death of a spouse" merited 100 such units. Using these weights, the cumulative impact of events experienced within a given time interval can then be calculated for each subject, by summing the Life Change Units appropriate for the events checked. This measure has been very widely employed in either a standard or modified form, and recent life changes have been found both to predict illness episodes in general and to be associated with the onset of specific diseases, including multiple sclerosis, cardiac arrest, rheumatoid arthritis, and tuberculosis (Dohrenwend & Dohrenwend, 1974; Johnson & Sarason, 1979; Rahe & Ranson 1978; Rabkin & Struening, 1976). The more life change experienced, the greater is the probability of illness onset and the more serious the illness is likely to be. This work has met with a number of criticisms, and it will be useful to review these since many reflect at a general level the methodological difficulties that are met with in psychosomatic studies of cancer.

A major problem is that, not only are the correlations between illness and measures of life change typically low (Holroyd, 1979; Horowitz, Schaeffer, Hiroto, Wilner, & Levin, 1977), but the interpretation of the relationship is problematic. Brown (1974) has pointed to three major sources of possible contamination. First, many studies in the area are retrospective, and illness could bias the way in which life events are reported. People's appraisal of their life style before illness may be distorted by their current state, or they may try to rationalize and justify their illness in terms of what has been happening to them previously. Second, illness can in some cases be itself a cause of life change. Even in its premorbid state, before specific symptoms are recognized, it could have a generalized physical and psychological effect. Problems within a marriage or at work, or changes in sleeping and other habits, might then be in fact an early outcome of the illness and only *seem* to antedate its onset. Both prospective and retrospective studies can be contaminated in this particular way, and both may be similarly vulnerable to a third difficulty of interpretation. The latter arises from the fact that a correlation between two variables can reflect an influence of another distinct variable on each independently, in the absence of a causal relationship between the original two, and life change and illness onset could vary in parallel because each is in its own right related to an external factor, such as anxiety. Yet another problem, and one not discussed by Brown, is the difficulty of distinguishing between an illness state and illness behavior. People do not always go to see the physician when ill, and it is sometimes other events that act as triggers for help-seeking. A person is more aware of symptoms when under stress, worries more about their implications, and is more likely to seek help and advice at such a time (Haney, 1977; Kasl & Cobb, 1966). Since in the great majority of cases illness is detected only when the person comes in with his or her symptoms, it follows that any observed relationship between life change and illness could reflect a variation in consultation rates, with the levels of illness actually experienced being a constant.

Other methodological discussions in the literature have been concerned with the kinds of life events and their psychological implications that are most relevant to the development of illness. The original questionnaire includes both undesirable and desirable events, but some studies have suggested that the former are the more significant (for example, Kellam, 1974). Another argument is that the significance of given events cannot be determined for the population as a whole, as assumed in the procedure of allocating standard weights to events to reflect the degree of readjustment they require. What is meaningful or meaningless, desirable or undesirable, for one person may not be so or may be so to a different degree for another (Redfield & Stone, 1979). Some researchers have thus based assessments of life change on the subject's own self-report of the disruptiveness of events (for example, Lundberg, Theorell, & Lind, 1975), rather than relying on ratings provided by a panel of judges. Brown and colleagues (1978) have adopted yet a different procedure, whereby the investigators evaluate the "upsettingness" of events reported, but within the context of the person's own values and life situation as these emerge in interview. In this way, it is hoped that full account can be taken of the person's subjective frame of reference, but without having to rely exclusively on self-report. Finally, one factor that might influence the impact of an event is the person's resources for coping. An event might have the same significance for two people in terms of the way it is evaluated and the readjustment needed, but one may be able to make the adjustment more easily than another, and several researchers have suggested that the person's capacity to master life changes will be an important variable when predicting the psychological and physical disturbance that will result (Dohrenwend & Dohrenwend, 1974; Mechanic, 1974; Rahe & Ranson, 1978). Kobasa (1982) has presented a description of the "hardy" personality, pointing to feelings of commitment, control and challenge as factors determining resistance to stress and consequent illness vulnerability.

With these last qualifications, the influence of personality is *implicitly* recognized as a causal factor in illness, mediating the impact of events. The person's own values and resources determine the way in which events are perceived and the ease with which adjustments are made, and vulnerability is thus determined by the interaction of external events and these internal factors. The theoretical construct that provides a unifying theme for this interaction is that of stress. Stress may be defined as a characteristic of a situation in which the demands placed on an organism are greater than the physical, psychological, and social resources that are available to meet these, and in any given situation stress can be primarily attributed to either the nature of these demands or to the resource capacity of the person, or to both in conjunction (McGrath, 1970). Stress has emotional consequences but also physical ones, and Hans Selye (1956) has described a sequence of distinct stages in the response to stress, referred to as the General Adaptation Syndrome. The first stage is that of alarm or emergency, during which there is a general increase in the activity of the pituitary-adrenocortical system. There follows a second stage of resistance, when the effects of the stress are successfully countered, but resistance to other stimuli may be decreased. Finally, if the stress is maintained there will be a breakdown in the process of adaptation as resources are exhausted and resistance fails. Selye originally conceived of the syndrome as a response to physically noxious events, but others have recently suggested that not only *can* the reaction occur as a response to psychological stress, but that the influence of physical agents is *generally* mediated by psychological factors (Mason, 1975). The model describes in far greater detail than is presented above the neuroendocrine and other physiological changes associated with stress, and these can provide the link between stress, of whatever origin, and susceptibility to illness. Stress might, first, enhance biological vulnerabilities that channel its effects so that the outcome is focused on the person's preexisting physical weaknesses (Bakal, 1979; Cannon, 1936; Seyle, 1956; Wolff, 1953). A second theory is that the characteristics of the stress response could in themselves determine the nature of the illness. While it is difficult to distinguish between different *emotions* at physiological level, patterns of autonomic and hormonal responses may be related to the characteristics of the stressor (Mason, 1975) and to the way in which the person copes in a stressful situation (Frankenhauser, 1976; Lacey, 1967; Obrist, 1976; Weiss, Glazer, & Pohorecky, 1976), and the maintenance of such responses over time could directly result in illness whose character is determined by the nature of the pattern. Third, exposure to stress might not in itself produce illness, but could bring about conditions under which illnesses could be easily established, as the ability to adapt becomes generally exhausted. Stress could affect the immunological response via the central nervous system and endocrine systems (Solomon, Amkraut, & Kasper, 1974), increasing the person's vulnerability and thus altering the balance between the person and any particular disease agents to which he or she is exposed (Cassel, 1974; Dubos, 1961). Possible mediating mechanisms between stress and cancer are discussed in a later section of this chapter.

Psychosocial Variables and Cancer: Retrospective Studies

Cancer, like heart disease, is an illness that researchers have singled out for particular attention. The existence of psychosomatic aspects of the disease was claimed before this century, and was it seems quite widely accepted (see Kowal, 1955). Bereavements and other trials, and the grief and anxiety they cause, were cited as precursors of the disease, and certain personality types were regarded as particularly vulnerable. Indeed, it was as early as the second century AD that Galen claimed that women of a "melancholic" temperament were more likely to get breast cancer than "sanguine" women. The clinical observations of those times have now been supplemented by a more systematic study of the relationship between psychological factors and the development of cancer, although truly controlled observation in this field remains an ideal and is difficult to achieve in practice. A great number of studies have been conducted, a variety of methods adopted, and diverse variables investigated. Several reviews of early and recent work have appeared and each of these has attempted its own organization and interpretation of the mass of data now available (Crisp, 1970; Fox, 1978; Goldfarb, Driesen, & Cole, 1967; Le Shan, 1960; Perrin & Pierce, 1959; Scurry & Levin, 1979). A summary of those studies that have focused on breast cancer patients is presented in Table 7-1.

Recent Life Events

Many writers have claimed that cancer patients typically experience a loss, separation, or frustration of life goals before the onset of their disease. Le Shan (1966) noted that cancer is statistically more common in women who are divorced or widowed, rather than in those who are stably married or single, and that the first symptom of cancer typically appears from six months to eight years after the loss of a significant relationship. Greene (1954, 1965, 1966) has similarly emphasized the role of life events and strain, noting a clustering of events such as family deaths, separations, and changes at work or home before the onset of leukemia. In relation to lung cancer, Kissen (1967) found a higher incidence of work, financial, and interpersonal difficulties in a group of cancer patients when compared with a group of controls, and a more recent study of lung cancer patients showed that they were more likely to have experienced a significant loss during the five years before developing the disease (Horne & Pickard, 1979). There are, however, a number of negative findings. Three studies have compared benign and malignant breast cases on life events, and have failed to find differences, or have found differences in the opposite direction to that predicted. Muslin, Gyarfas, and Pieper (1966) found no difference between the two groups in separation experiences during the three years before diagnosis; Greer and Morris (1975) could detect no significant differences between breast patients with benign and malignant lesions on a measure of life stress; and Schonfield (1975) found that it was benign patients who had the higher total life event scores, although the groups were not significantly different on those items that related specifically to loss. It is notable that the studies with negative findings quoted above all involve breast patients, and it is possible that etiological factors are different depending on the site of a cancer. Stephenson and Grace (1954), for example, found that patients with cervical cancer had higher incidences of divorce and desertion than women with cancer at other sites. Also, in the three studies cited, the control group comprised patients who had benign breast lesions, and it may be that the life stress factors that contribute to breast cancer are implicated in other breast disease as well. Yet another discriminating factor may be the fact that these studies employed relatively structured measures of change, such as the Schedule of Recent Experience. This approach avoids the interview bias that might conceivably arise from a prediction of greater losses in cancer patients, but is also less sensitive to factors such as desirability of events and their personal significance for the person concerned. Thus, the occurrence of a loss or

Table 7-1. Studies of Personality and Life History Variables in Breast Cancer Patients

Study	Groups Investigated	Stage of Assessment	Principle Findings
Tarlau and Smalheiser, 1951	Breast cancer Cervical cancer No control	Postdiagnosis	A pattern of mother dominance and rejection of the feminine role in both cancer groups. Negative attitudes toward sexuality, though a superficial adjustment in the case of breast cancer patients.
Bacon et al., 1952	Breast cancer No control	Postdiagnosis	Unresolved conflict with the mother, masochism, inhibited sexuality, inhibited motherhood, inability to discharge anger.
Reznikoff, 1955	Breast cancer Benign breast disease Control group of well women	Prediagnosis	A greater likelihood of death of a sibling at birth or in infancy in the cancer group, and excessive responsibility in childhood. Negative feelings toward pregnancy and birth, and disturbances in feminine identification.
Wheeler and Caldwell, 1955	Breast cancer Cervical cancer Control group of hospital patients	Postdiagnosis	A more disturbed and insecure background for cervical but not breast cancer patients. Negative feelings toward heterosexual relations in both cancer groups.
Muslin et al., 1966	Breast cancer Benign breast disease	Prediagnosis	No differences in early or recent separation experiences.
Coppen and Metcalfe, 1964	Breast ($n=32$) and other cancers ($n=15$) Control group of gynecological and other surgical patients	Postdiagnosis	Higher extroversion for breast cancer patients. No difference in neuroticism.
Greer and Morris, 1975	Breast cancer Benign breast disease	Prediagnosis	No differences in life stress, level of hostility, extroversion, or depression. Abnormal release of emotion, especially anger.
Schonfield, 1975	Breast cancer Benign breast disease	Prediagnosis	No differences in depression and well-being, or losses and separation. Indeed, the benign group had the higher life change units.

frustration that was of primary psychological importance might not be appropriately differentiated from other occurrences, and the latter could mask the impact of the former. Finally, one recent study of the relationship between bereavement and cancer has claimed to find little evidence of a link (Jones, Goldblatt, & Leon, 1984). Using census data from 1971-1975, registrations of cancer after the death of a spouse in this period were not significantly increased, and there was only a slight suggestion of increased mortality from cancer. However, a longer follow-up would be required to test the hypothesis adequately, since it may well take some time for a cancer to develop and be detected and, indeed, there was greater evidence of an increase in cancer among an incomplete cohort of women who had lost their husbands before 1966.

Early Experience

In the cancer literature there is as much emphasis placed on early as on recent life experience. Cancer patients, it is claimed, are more likely to have suffered separation or some other crisis as a child, or to have had a conflictful relationship with one or other parent. Le Shan describe a pattern of unresolved tensions with parents, possibly associated with early life crisis (Le Shan, 1966; Le Shan & Worthington, 1956); Kissen (1967) observed that childhood relationships were distorted in both a lung cancer and psychosomatic group; and Bahnson (1969), comparing cancer patients with a myocardial infarction group, found that the former thought of their parents as having been more neglecting. Studies with breast cancer patients have produced similar findings. Wheeler and Caldwell (1955) noted a generally more disturbed and insecure background in patients with both breast and cervical cancer when they were children, and Reznikoff (1955), comparing breast cancer patients with a benign control group and with a group free from pathology, noted that the former were more likely to have experienced the death of a sibling in infancy and to have had to assume greater responsibility as a child. Bacon and colleagues (1952) point to an unresolved conflict with the mother in particular as a predisposing factor, at least with regard to the younger breast cancer patient, and Tarlau and Smalheiser (1951) similarly talk of mother dominance resulting in a rejection of the feminine role.

Personality

Cancer patients are often characterized as being negative in their attitudes toward themselves. They have been described as self-critical (Le Shan, 1966; Le Shan & Worthington, 1956) and self-sacrificing (Schmale & Iker, 1966). Some studies have suggested that they are relatively low in neuroticism and emotional responsivity (for example Kissen, 1963) and others that they show little anger and hostility (Le Shan & Worthington, 1956). Such findings would in many circumstances be interpreted as an indication of good adjustment and emotional stability, but in this context they are more often regarded as resulting from poor emotional *discharge*, the assumption being that anxiety and anger are experienced but not expressed. This interpretation is supported by studies that have found higher levels of denial and repression in cancer patients (Abse et al., 1974;

Bahnson & Bahnson, 1966; Dattore, Shontz, & Goyne, 1980). Perhaps the most frequently cited correlates of the disease are a clustering of negative mood states, all relating to depression. It is many centuries since Galen first made the claim of an association between melancholia and cancer, and current descriptions of the cancer patient still refer to despair and hopelessness (Bahnson, 1969; Greene, 1966; Le Shan, 1966; Schmale, 1966). Indeed, Schmale and Iker (1971) were able to make a better than chance prediction of those women from a group of patients suspected of cervical cancer who would, in fact, be found to have the disease, on the basis of their hopelessness as a reaction to life stress. Despair and hopelessness reflect an appraisal of the present as lacking in meaning, and of the future as without promise, but the psychological orientation determining this kind of appraisal may be rooted in the past. Both Le Shan (1966) and Bahnson (1969) talk of the significance of a later loss or frustration *in the context* of earlier losses or unsatisfactory relationships; these can have a sensitizing effect, and enhance vulnerability to later adversity. Thus, early experience influences personality which, in turn, can modify the impact of more recent life events.

Studies of breast cancer patients support some but not all of these conclusions with regard to personality. They have been described as self-sacrificing (Bacon et al., 1952), as rejecting their feminine role (Tarlau & Smalheiser, 1951), and as having both sexual and general role difficulties (Reznikoff, 1955). It is sometimes claimed that breast cancer patients are characterized by extroversion, with a positive finding in a study by Coppen and Metcalfe (1963) and some supportive evidence from Hagnell (1966). Greer and Morris, however, found no evidence of such a difference when comparing patients with benign and malignant breast lesions (1975). Although differences on neuroticism, depression or general well-being have not been found (Coppen & Metcalfe, 1963; Greer & Morris, 1975; Schonfield, 1975), there is some evidence of a repression or suppression of anger and hostility (Bacon et al., 1972; Greer & Morris, 1975; Schonfield, 1975). Indeed, in one recent study it was possible to differentiate before biopsy, at a significant statistical level, women who had malignant tumors on the basis of their suppression of anxiety, and their apparent optimism and self-sufficiency (Wirsching, Stierlin, Hoffmann, Weber, & Wirsching, 1982). These characteristics were interpreted as defense mechanisms employed to cope with the current stressful situation, and functioning as a reaction against underlying anxiety, despair, and helplessness. The description of an overtly helpless and hopeless, or despairing, personality does not, however, feature much in descriptions of the patient with breast cancer.

Summary of Findings

The general picture of the cancer patient that emerges, then, is of someone who has had a disturbed childhood; has poor outlets for emotional discharge, and reacts to difficulties with despair and hopelessness. In the case of specific cancers the pattern might be somewhat different. For example, conflicts about gender role and sexuality are cited in the breast cancer literature, but are not commonly attributed to cancer patients in general, while the reverse is true of despair and hopelessness. These comments must, however, be regarded as speculative because of the absence of research that has systematically compared one group of cancer patients with another, and because the methodological and substantive differences in studies that have each looked at cancer in one site outlaw a direct comparison between these. Second, not only might personality and life history profiles be different according to the type of cancer, but there could well be differences within each group depending on the characteristics of the disease. In one study (Becker, 1979), younger breast cancer patients showed a pattern of a cold and distrustful family atmosphere, early loss, an achieving personality, a denial of the traditional female role, and low sexuality. This pattern was absent in those women who had developed cancer later in life.

Methodological Criticisms and Prospective Studies

There are a variety of criticisms that can be aimed at these kinds of retrospective studies, criticisms of which the researchers themselves are usually well aware. In the case of any single study that claims to offer support for a psychosomatic hypothesis, the skeptic is generally able to point to one or more of several alternative interpretations.

1. Because of the quantity of speculation and claims that point to a psychosomatic origin of cancer, most researchers would *expect* to find differences in the cancer group. They would probably not be carrying out the investigation if they did not believe in at least the plausibility of the hypothesis that such differences do exist. These expectations can easily influence any data gathered in interview and the way in which they are interpreted (Le Shan, 1960). This particular difficulty of interpretation is compounded in studies that employ no control group, and this is true of many studies in the area (for example, Bacon et al., 1952; Greene, 1954, 1956). Without a control group, there can be no base-line with reference to which conclusions about the cancer groups may be drawn, and the preconceptions of the investigator might lead to an overemphasis on characteristics of the cancer group that are, in fact, representative of the general population. In order to avoid biases in both the collection and interpretation of data, some researchers have tried to keep themselves ignorant of patients' diagnoses until after interview, but ignorance may be difficult to maintain given that subjects who themselves know or suspect their diagnosis can provide clues or direct information about this (Abse et al., 1974). A second possible solution is to minimize the interaction between the investigator and the subject, and hence any unintentional influence of the former's expectations, by using tests, inventories, questionnaires or interviews that have a clear structure and standardized format. However, the advantages of this approach may in some circumstances be outweighed by its disadvantages. Where patients are reticent and anxious, the researcher may feel that meaningful information *can* only be obtained in the context of a rapport between himself or herself and the patient, and where there is a willingness to let the assessment be guided by the patient's own individual style and behavior.

2. Different investigations have used a variety of groups for comparison with cancer patients. Where the study involves cancer at a particular site, then a common strategy is to use, as a control, patients who have some nonmalignant disease at the same site. When studying lung cancer patients, comparison may be made with patients suffering from other chest disorders such as tuberculosis (Abse et al., 1974; Booth, 1964; Kissen et al., 1969), while patients with breast cancer are frequently compared with others who have benign breast disease (Greer & Morris, 1975; Reznikoff, 1955; Schonfield, 1975). Often, the control group comprises patients with a variety of nonmalignant conditions, whether the cancer group is heterogeneous or comprises patients with cancer at one site only (Coppen & Metcalfe, 1963; Dattore et al., 1980; Wheeler & Caldwell, 1955). Alternatively, the control group chosen may be free of all apparent pathology (Le Shan & Worthington, 1956; Reznikoff, 1955). The nature of the control group or groups employed obviously determines the range of conclusions that can be legitimately drawn. Only where illness is involved can it be concluded that any differences between this and a cancer group are related specifically to cancer as opposed to pathology in general. Schmale (1969) does in fact argue that helplessness and hopelessness are not features only of the cancer patient's history and personality but factors common in the etiology of many diseases: "From our studies it is now evident that there is nothing specific about the psychological setting for the patient with cancer that differentiates him from patients who develop other diseases. The failure of repressions, denial and inhibition as defenses, the loss of sources of object or self-gratification, the feelings of depression and no motivation to change things are all part of the setting in which disease, including cancer, has its onset." Greene (1965, p. 629–630) similarly argues that a setting of loss and unsuccessful coping, characterized by grief and depression, can lead to the manifestation of or relapse into illness in many varied diseases.

3. Yet another variation between studies that has implications for the interpretation of findings is the stage at which patients are assessed. Some researchers have interviewed patients before their illness has been diagnosed (Greer & Morris, 1975; Muslin et al., 1966; Reznikoff, 1955; Schmale & Iker, 1971), separating benign from malignant cases after the diagnosis has been made. At the other extreme, studies have included patients seen many years after the detection and treatment of their cancer, and even patients with advanced disease (Le Shan & Worthington, 1956; Tarlau & Smalheiser, 1951; Wheeler & Caldwell, 1955). More commonly, the assessment takes place during or just after treatment. Where the diagnosis has already been made, it is possible that patients' emotionality or defensiveness, or their general way of viewing themselves and the world, arises from an awareness of cancer and the fact of its treatment. This is a confounding factor affecting all retrospective studies and has already been mentioned in the context of life events and general illnesses. Feelings of despair and hopelessness, defenses such as denial, and the suppression of hostility, are commonly cited as an outcome of the illness, and the observation of these characteristics in cancer patients by no means implies that these are traits that preexisted the illness. In other words, these characteristics of cancer patients observed after the illness have been discovered can be interpreted either as states related to their

current situation or as long-term traits and dispositions. It is more difficult, but not impossible, to interpret reports of early disturbance and intrafamilial tension in cancer patients in the same way: it could be argued that awareness of the disease might bias patients' reports and memories of their early experience (Greene, 1966). From the vulnerable position of being a cancer patient, not only the future but also the past may be judged as less secure.

There are two principal approaches to controlling for this kind of confounding. The first is to use as a control group patients whose illness is of a similar degree of severity, a recommendation made by Perrin and Pierce (1959). Patients with heart conditions have been suggested as suitable candidates by Le Shan (1960) and have been employed by Bahnson and Bahnson (1966), but it cannot be claimed that the stresses involved in this or any other illness are identical with regard to its implications for future health or for treatment. The second approach is to assess patients before the diagnosis is made, as some researchers have done. This reduces but does not avoid difficulties of interpretation, since in many cases patients may have suspicions of their diagnosis on the basis of the nature and severity of their symptoms, an "unconscious" awareness of disease (Grinker, 1966), their family history, or some preliminary feedback from their general practitioner (Chesser & Anderson, 1975). The only way of completely avoiding the difficulty is to carry out prospective studies in which initially healthy people are interviewed and tested, and to use these data to compare those who subsequently develop cancer with those who escape the disease. There are now a number of such prospective studies in the literature. One is that of Hagnell (1966), for which 2,500 people were followed up over a period of twenty years. The women who later contracted cancer were found to have had higher scores, at the earlier assessment, on a personality dimension known as "substability." This is said to be related to extroversion, and comprises characteristics such a warmth, naivety, industriousness, sociability, and a tendency toward personal relationships. They were also depressive in their personality type. In another study, more than 1,300 inhabitants of a Yugoslavian town were assessed on a questionnaire oriented toward those psychological factors thought to be associated with disease. Ten years later, it was found that the items on the questionnaire discriminated successfully between people who had later developed illness and those without a diagnosis, and between cancer patients and those who developed other internal diseases (Grossarth-Maticek, 1980, 1983). Those who developed cancer were characterized as having high emotional needs, the experience of loss or withdrawal of the object of these needs, and a reaction of helplessness and depression. This pattern contrasted with that of cardiovascular patients whose needs were frustrated by others and the environment and who reacted to this with chronic irritation and anger. Third, in a study by Bieliauskas (see Bahnson, 1980), those of a group of over 2,000 subjects who had died of cancer were shown to have higher scores on the depression scale of the Minnesota Multiphasic Personality Inventory (MMPI), administered 17 years previously. A finding inconsistent with this and other findings is that of Dattore and colleagues (1980), who compared the premorbid scores of 200 cancer and noncancer patients in a Veterans Administration hospital, on the MMPI, and found higher repression but *lower* depression scores for the cancer group. Most prospective studies have been concerned with personality and its relationship to cancer, but one study has focused on early experience and family relationships (Thomas, Duszynski, & Shaffer, 1979). A group of more than 1300 medical students have now been followed up for a number of years, and those of the group who were later to develop either cancer or mental illness, or to commit suicide, were more likely on their initial assessment of family attitudes to have claimed a lack of closeness to their parents, their father in particular. This was not true of those who were later to develop hypertension or coronary heart disease.

Even prospective studies, however, do not allow for perfect control. There are three further explanations for a relationship between life experiences and personality on the one hand and cancer, on the other, which they do not exclude:

4. The former could be an *outcome* of cancer, as an effect of the disease process at a stage before its discovery. A tumor may be present many years before it is detected, and even in this latent state the disease could have a general impact on lifestyle and well-being (Joynt, 1974; Kerr, Schapira, & Roth, 1969; Whitlock & Siskind, 1979).

5. The relationship between psychological variables and cancer could be due to the conjoint influence of a demographic variable such as age or class, in which case there is no causal relationship, or psychological factors could determine exposure to other environmental or behavioral ones that themselves cause cancer, in which case the causal relationship is an indirect one only. Finally, life experiences and personality could affect not the development of the illness itself but the person's reaction to symptoms. As argued earlier, life stress and emotional difficulties may bring the patient to the physician to consult about symptoms which might not otherwise command attention (Haney, 1977; Kasl & Cobb, 1966). Some cases of cancer are slow in their development and may be more quickly detected in people who have some additional incentive to consult. These would then be overrepresented in the numbers of those whose cancer has been *diagnosed*, and the incidence figures would be correspondingly biased.

In summary, an observed association between cancer and psychological variables does not necessarily imply that the latter predispose the person to the former. In any particular case, the direction of the causal relationship could, arguably, be the reverse of that assumed, or variables other than these could determine the association. It must also be acknowledged that many studies that have looked for an association have failed to find this (Fox, 1978); such inconsistencies may result from differences in the variables selected, methods of assessment, and the groups studied, and there is a great need in this area for faithful replications of those studies that have produced positive results and an elucidation of their defining characteristics. In our opinion, nevertheless, it would be foolish at this stage to "throw the baby out with the bath water" in an excess of methodological zeal. When the conclusions of so many studies with different designs and weaknesses point in the same direction, an outright rejection of this evidence may prove to be premature. Furthermore, animal investigations provide some support for the hypothesis of a causal relationship between psychosocial-stress factors and cancer, and such studies, being experimental in nature, obviate the difficulties of interpretation implicit in studies with human subjects. While it is true that results here too are sometimes inconsistent, there is also some indication of certain key criteria that determine whether or not an effect is observed. These include the kind of stress created and the possibility of coping allowed. Thus Sklar and Anisman (1979) found that mice exposed to electric shock showed earlier tumor appearance, larger tumor size, and decreased survival following cell transplantation. However, this occurred only if the shock was inescapable, and did not occur in those mice (with whom the former were yoked) who had the possibility of escaping shock. Also, chronic as opposed to acute shock exposure seemed to abrogate the effects of stress. Thus, control and adaptation are two modulating factors in this context, and it is only in their absence that stress had the effect of enhancing tumor growth. With a greater attention to such factors, it may be possible to resolve some of the inconsistencies and controversies that beset human studies.

New Directions

Many have balked at accepting an influence of psychological factors on cancer due in part to the mind-body dualism which has prevailed until recently within this culture and which has perhaps been especially prevalent in medical circles. There is, however, no need to invoke metaphysical explanations for a link, and two possible candidates for this role are the neuroendocrine system and cell-mediated immunity.

Cell-Mediated Immunity

There is now a considerable body of evidence that cell-mediated immunity involving thymic dependent lymphocytes, the monocyte macrophage series of cells, and natural killer cells may influence the development and progression of cancer. This work holds good for most experimental carcinogen-induced tumors, but it must be acknowledged that there is still only indirect evidence that cell-mediated immunity is of clinical relevance in the evolution and progression of cancer in humans. Studies of the effects of stress on immunity have shown immunosuppression in both animals and humans. In rats, for example, exposure to uncontrollable shock has been found to depress lymphocyte proliferations in response to mitogens (Laudenslayer, Ryan, Drugan, Hysor, & Maier, 1983). In humans, one study has shown depressed lymphocyte function six weeks after bereavement (Barthrop, Lazarus, Luckhurst, Kiluh, & Penny, 1977) and the prospective Yugoslavian study referred to earlier found that psychosocial stress was associated with a low lymphocyte functioning (Grossarth-Matick, Kanazier, Vetter, & Schmidt, 1983). A recent and interesting study by Kiecolt-Glaser, Garner, Speicher, Penn, Holliday, and Glaser (1984) observed medical students before and during their final examinations. The latter produced a decline in natural killer cells, and levels of these were related also to loneliness and life events assessed by questionnaire.

Neuroendocrine Pathways

Stress can influence levels of circulating hormones, and these in turn may affect immunologic surveillance. Cortisol, βestradiol, and testosterone are the three hormones that have been most carefully studied in their relationship to the mechanism of cell-mediated immunity, with the expression of immunity being studied either by nonspecific or specific delayed cutaneous hypersensitivity reactions that involve interactions between lymphocytes and macrophages. In addition, the specific function of the monocyte macrophage system of cells has also been studied in relation to administered hormones or following the reduction of endogenous hormone levels by castration. In general, cortisol depresses all the variables of cell-mediated immunity that have been studied, whereas the estrogens and androgens have a variable effect depending on which group of cells is studied. In relation to factors that might be specifically involved in the development of breast cancer, Bulbrook and Hayward (1967) were perhaps the first to demonstrate that hormone levels in the blood may determine the risk of a woman developing carcinoma of the breast. In their classic prospective study carried out on the island of Guernsey, they collected urine from all the women at risk of developing breast cancer and stored it up for 15 years. During this period of observation a large number of women on the island developed the disease and, following its detection, their stored sample of urine was analyzed for hormone metabolites and compared with other stored specimens of urine from matched control patients who had not yet developed the disease. Significant differences in androgen and corticosteroid metabolites were detected between the two populations. Apart from this, there is a considerable body of evidence to suggest that luteal phase insufficiency, whereby the breast duct epithelium is exposed to high levels of estrogen in the latter part of each menstrual cycle in the absence of the modulating effect of progesterone produced by the corpus luteum, may contribute to the development of breast cancer.

For these reasons any factors that influence the production of the trophic hormones from the pituitary may indirectly contribute to the development of breast cancer. Thus, follicular-stimulating hormone and luteinizing hormone control the development of the ovarian follicle and corpus luteum, whereas ACTH influences the production of corticosteroids from the adrenal gland, some of which can be metabolized into estrogenic compounds. In addition, the hormone prolactin, which is also produced in the anterior pituitary gland, has a direct influence on the development and proliferation of the lactiferous ducts and lobules within the breast. Prolactin has certainly been implicated in the development of experimental rat mammary gland tumors, although its role in human breast cancer remains uncertain. The activity of the anterior pituitary gland is controlled from the hypothalamus via a portal system of vessels transmitting releasing factors for ACTH, FSH, LH, and prolactin. The hypothalamus in its turn is linked via the limbic system to the thalamus and cerebral cortex. Thus, stress could arguably influence the behavior of breast duct epithelium either directly or indirectly via the production of adrenal and ovarian hormones.

There is, in conclusion, a distinct possibility of a convergence between two areas of research hitherto unrelated: one being the influence of personality and stress on disease, and the other being immunologic and endocrine studies. All disease is multifactorial—involving genetic, hormonal, neurochemical, immunological, and emotional factors. The interactions between these are difficult to disentangle, and the mediating mechanisms suggested are at present speculative and hypothetical. The study of these relationships is, however, attracting increasing interest and offers the prospect of a novel perspective on an understanding of disease. A more detailed review of research within the expanding field of psychoimmunoneurology is presented by Ader (1981).

A related research question in future years is likely to be that of the relationship between psychosocial variables and the *outcome* of cancer. Psychological variables may not only influence patients' adjustment to their illness and recovery after treatment (Schonfield, 1972) but might also affect survival. William Parker in the Nineteenth century claimed that patients get well by "self-denial, perseverance, pluck and determination" (Kowal, 1955), and various writers since then have suggested that the relief of psychological symptoms might prolong the patient's life (for example, Prendergrass, 1965). There are still relatively few empirical studies of this question. One of the earliest was that of Blumberg, West, and Ellis (1954), who used the MMPI to assess patients with inoperable tumors and concluded that those with more slowly growing cancers were able to avoid or reduce stress, whether by normal activity or defensive means. Krasnoff (1959), however, failed to replicate these findings in a study of patients with malignant melanoma. The area is bedevilled with such inconsistent results. Weisman and Worden (1977) found that longer term survivors were less distressed, regarded their physician as helpful, complained less, and coped better. However, in a study of patients with metastatic breast cancer (Derogatis, Abeloff, & Melisaratos, 1979), survival was found to be associated with a *poorer* psychological adjustment to illness. Survivors showed higher hostility, anxiety, and psychoticism, and negative mood states. In a similar vein, Stavraky, Buck, Lott, and Wanklin (1968) noted that patients with a favorable outcome were more hostile than those with an unfavorable outcome, and it was their scores that were more similar to those of a control group without cancer. This suggests the hypothesis that patients who are apparently well-adjusted may be showing suppression of feeling. The findings of a recent study by Greer and colleagues (1979) echo some but not all of these findings. Recurrence-free survival seemed more likely where patients showed a "fighting spirit." This was described as an optimistic attitude, a search for information about their condition, and a strong motivation to overcome it. This is not the same as hostility, but both orientations reflect an acknowledgment of the threat in the situation and an impulse to confront and overcome this. An attitude of helplessness and hopelessness was associated with earlier recurrence, as was stoic acceptance of the diagnosis. Defensiveness in the form of a denial of the diagnosis and its significance had favorable implications for outcome, and this parallels Blumberg's findings. The study has been criticized for its small sample size, and the possibility that subgroups might differ in the clinical stage of their disease, and it is now being replicated.

Obviously, there is as yet no pattern of results consistent across studies, and there is a need for more sophisticated measurement of both psychological and biological variables and for distinction to be made between and within different kinds of cancer. Furthermore, if patients' emotional distress and way of coping with the illness were related to length of survival, then there would remain the question of whether tumor growth and the process of dissemination were themselves affected, or whether the effect was more superficial in terms of duration of life, with the disease state a constant.

Summary

Recent life events involving change and disruption seem to increase vulnerability to illness, and stress could theoretically either enhance existing physiological weaknesses, or give rise to specific illnesses depending on the pattern of chronic reactions that it evokes, or weaken resistance to infection and other attacks. Retrospective studies of cancer patients have investigated their recent life events, early experiences, and personality. Cancer patients in general are more likely to have had a disturbed childhood, to be inhibited in expressing their emotions, and to react to setbacks with despair and hopelessness. There are many criticisms that can be made of these studies. Prospective studies obviate some but not all of these, and they too indicate loss, depression, helplessness, and childhood difficulties as predisposing factors. Experimental studies with animals are less open to ambiguities of interpretation, although they obviously cannot replicate the experiences and responses of human subjects. Here, there is evidence that stress can enhance tumor growth, but only in the absence of possibilities of controlling and adapting to the stressor. This latter qualification suggests hypotheses that might fruitfully be explored in the human context.

There are two pathways that are obvious candidates when considering the mediation between psychosocial factors and the etiology of cancer. It seems, first, that stress can affect cell-mediated immunity, and, second, that hormones whose levels are influenced by stress can affect immunologic surveillance. Discussions of the specific mechanisms that might be involved are still speculative, but the field of psychoneuroimmunology offers exciting prospects for interdisciplinary research in the future.

8

Implications for the Care of the Breast Cancer Patient

A Shift in Emphasis

Clinicians' increasing interest over the last decade in psychological aspects of breast cancer reflects a conceptual shift in our model of the disease itself. It is now more than one hundred years ago that Dr. Halsted from the Johns Hopkins Hospital, Baltimore, described the classic radical mastectomy, an operation that was developed as a result of certain firmly held assumptions about the behavior of the disease. The viewpoint in retrospect appears extremely mechanistic. The cancer was believed to arise as a single focus within the breast, enlarging with time and spreading continuously along the lymphatics. It was assumed that the disease was arrested in the axillary lymph nodes, and these were looked on as filters. With the passage of time, it was thought, the filters became exhausted. The cancer continued to spread through the efferent lymphatics along fascial planes, and, after penetrating the deep fascia vital organs such as the liver, it finally infiltrated brain and bone marrow. With this view, it seemed entirely plausible that a simple mastectomy would only cure those women whose disease was confined to the breast, and that, to improve the cure rate, the tissue removed had to be extended. Furthermore, to avoid transecting the lymphatics and spilling cancer cells in the operative field, this operation had to be done *en bloc*. Thus, the classic Halsted radical mastectomy involved removal of the breast, the pectoralis major, pectoralis minor, and the axillary lymphatic tissue in continuity.

   In spite of recognition in the 1930s and 1940s of the failure of this approach to achieve a cure, the fundamental assumptions were not questioned. Instead, surgeons and radiotherapists assumed that the area treated was not large enough. During a short but tragic period in the history of the disease, some surgeons went as far as to perform forequarter amputation, removing the arm in continuity with the breast and lymphatic tissue. Other surgeons extended the operation into the neck, taking out the cervical lymph nodes, while others carried out an extended radical mastectomy, which involved dissecting out the lymphatics from within the mediastinum. As an alternative approach, radiotherapists felt that they could increase the field of treatment by adding a course of radical radiotherapy to the radical operation. None of these approaches in fact improved survival rates, although all of them increased the morbidity of the procedure, leading to greater mutilation and a high incidence of massive lymphoedema of the arm. As a small compensation, though, there was a reduction in the incidence of *local* recurrence.

Throughout this time, little thought was given to the quality of the patient's life or the psychological impact of these invasive procedures, because the surgeons and radiotherapists alike were secure in their conviction that they were doing their very best to save patients' lives, and all other effects of treatment were peripheral to this priority. Over the last 10 years, however, a conceptual revolution has occurred, and the current prevailing model of the disease is a "deterministic" one. It is now widely accepted that the outcome of treatment for early breast cancer is predetermined by the extent of micrometastases present at the time of diagnosis and not by the extent of local therapy. Furthermore, it is now thought that involvement of the axillary lymph nodes, rather than being a determinant of outcome, is merely symptomatic of the residual tumor burden following local therapy. As a result of these changes in attitude, the role of surgery and radiotherapy has been redefined. Surgeons and radiotherapists alike would readily admit that if they cure the patient it is luck rather than skill, with the successful outcome largely dependent on the unknown biological properties of the cancer. In these circumstances the major contribution of mastectomy and radiotherapy should be looked on as palliative. They cannot be regarded as curative, although they do play an important role in the control of local disease. This conclusion has led many to turn to adjuvant systemic therapy as the hope for the future, recognizing that improvements in survival are unlikely without some treatment of this kind. It is somewhat alarming, though, that their use has become therapeutic dogma in many parts of the world, in view of the unquestionably severe side effects of many of these agents. While a new conceptual rationale holds that adjuvant chemotherapy ought to work, that is a long way from having demonstrated that it truly does work, and this treatment is still experimental. Clinicians today, therefore, have to face the fact that much of their treatment is limited in its effectiveness and are giving more serious consideration to the morbidity associated with mastectomy, radiotherapy, and chemotherapy. Most treatment involves some cost, whether physical or psychological, and the ethical basis for the treatment of cancer should be a clear judgment that the benefits achieved outweigh the suffering entailed (Greer, 1984). The patient's quality of life should be an issue even where a treatment has been demonstrated to be effective, and it should assume an even greater importance where the aim of the treatment is palliative or its efficiency is in doubt.

Reducing the Stress of Breast Cancer

The clinician's role is a stressful one, offering treatments which he knows can cure no more than a minority of patients and deciding between treatment alternatives whose merits have, in some cases, yet to be established. He needs courage to overcome the frustrations of this situation and to meet its challenges. He needs courage similarly if he is to maintain an open and supportive relationship with the patient, even where he knows that there is little he can do for her by way of his medical skills. Only then can he act as the "sustaining presence" that can give her, in turn, the courage to face the difficulties that she faces (Shelp, 1984). The situation from the point of view of both physician and patient challenges two basic myths to which we irrationally cling and from which we habitually derive much of our strength. Unconsciously, if not consciously, we feel that anything can be achieved as long as we try hard enough or want it badly enough, and we regard death as something that comes to other people, or to ourselves, but in some far distant future. An illness like cancer cuts through these illusions of omnipotence and immortality, and courage is needed to carry on without them, and somehow not only to accept but also to transcend our limitations. Shelp argues that illness provides opportunities for growth on the part of both physician and patient. It provides "a context in which the nature of the human condition can be learned and the character necessary to negotiate reality can be developed" (1984, p. 359). This is of course an ideal as opposed to a description of what actually occurs. Some clinicians feel that these issues lie beyond the legitimate boundary of their role; they see themselves as "getting on with the job" and let the patient "do her own adjusting." Others take a similar stance in practice, but do so in order to manage their own stress in the situation rather than because their definition of their role prescribes it. To do more, they may argue, would be to run the risk of being overwhelmed. They may feel also that they lack the empathy and interpersonal skills that would be required by a more active concern with the patient's psychological needs. Much of the responsibility for fostering such attitudes, resources, and skills lies with the medical schools, in providing the relevant teaching and experience and treating this as a valued component of the curriculum. It is at this stage that the student acquires habits and ways of thinking that may influence his or her practice throughout a career. The responsibility lies also with the social scientists who contribute to such courses, to ensure that what they teach is really relevant to a practicing physician's needs. Knowledge about the origins of the health service or the psychology of learning may have an erudite appeal, but does not have the impact on *practice* that can be achieved by role play, discussion, and other exercises that focus directly on the physician-patient relationship and the issues pertinent to this.

Meanwhile, some additional provision needs to be made if patients' problems are to be coped with adequately. The recent introduction of specialist nurses or mastectomy counselors is, therefore, very welcome. Ideally, the nurse might coordinate activity and act as a liaison officer within a team headed by a surgeon. This team would comprise radiotherapists and a medical oncologist, and would be supported by a psychiatrist or psychologist and by community-based specialists for secondary referral. Innovations such as this, however, deserve careful planning and evaluation. For example, one issue that needs to be resolved is the extent to which the nurse can independently help patients to adjust psychologically. Must her role be limited to monitoring patients and detecting needs, with the benefits of her intervention being dependent on her ability then to refer to some other agency? Or can she actively deal with patients' concerns and counsel in a way that fosters good coping and prevents significant problems from arising? If the latter is the goal, then nurses should be provided with a formal training in counseling and stress management to equip them for this. The role of the nurse in this context should become more clearly defined over the next decade, and it would be helpful to compare empirically the outcomes of different sorts of approaches on emotional well-being and morbidity, in addition to evaluating interventions in isolation. Whether or not psychological support can, apart from reducing the stressfulness of the illness and its treatment, influence the biological outcome of the disease, is a separate though related question. There is some suggestion within the literature that psychosocial interventions might influence survival, and the hypothesis certainly merits a scientific evaluation.

Breast cancer causes concern not only to the patient who has the disease, but also among the general public, and one of the goals of health education should be to counter inappropriate perceptions of the disease and of the woman's vulnerability to it. Appeals that confine themselves to preaching that early diagnosis saves lives, and to advocating breast self-examination and prompt consultation, are tackling only part of the problem. There are still many misconceptions and irrational fears about cancer, and these should be targets for change, not only because they can prevent desirable behaviors, but also because they can cause anxiety where none, or anxiety to a lesser degree, is justified. Thus, women with cyclical breast pain need to be reassured that this is not commonly a symptom of cancer and that, furthermore, breast cancer rarely occurs before the age of 30, and women within the cancer age group can be offered the reassurance that the majority of breast lumps are, in fact, benign. At the moment, many women who discover a breast symptom assume that this is more likely than not to mean cancer, and, even if they are later informed that it is not, the foreboding experienced in the interim could have a profound effect on their view of their lives and on their relationships. Messages should, therefore, be oriented toward reassurance as much as toward indicating risk and, as with any appeal whatever its import, care must be taken not to arouse greater anxiety than is warranted by the health gains that can actually be achieved. In this area, as in others, it is imperative that we have empirical studies to monitor the outcomes of our efforts and that these should include detrimental and unintended outcomes, as well as those that are the avowed goal of the intervention.

Alternative Treatments and Clinical Trials

There is much interest at present in developing forms of treatment for breast cancer that are psychologically and physically acceptable to patients, and a critical issue here is whether these offer equivalent benefits to the patient in terms of dealing with the cancer. At the same time, new developments could in the future reduce the chance of recurrence, providing treatments that might be more acceptable by virtue of their enhanced benefits rather than by reducing morbidity. The merits of these alternatives can only be assessed by controlled clinical trials, without which assumptions and dogma may remain unchallenged.

For nearly 100 years, progress in the management of breast cancer had been held back by a rigid adherence to a mechanistic concept of the disease that resulted in widespread adoption of radical surgery and radical radiotherapy. The first randomized clinical trials of treatment for early breast cancer were introduced in the mid-1950s, and, in retrospect, they can be looked on as the beginning of the challenge to orthodox beliefs about the disease. The net result of the clinical trials conducted over the last 20 years has been an effective refutation of the mechanistic (Halstedian) hypothesis, and this has given rise to a new and more attractive biological, deterministic model. The role of local therapy has been redefined in terms of local control, and, as already described, modest benefits can be attributed to the early results of trials of systemic therapy.

There are currently two main directions in which improvements in therapy are being sought. On the one hand, trials of breast conservation will determine whether preserving the breast can achieve the same outcome as mastectomy, using local control and survival rates as the endpoints. On the other hand, different trials are exploring alternative strategies for systemic therapy following local therapy, comparing the outcome of "soft" options with that of conventional, aggressive chemotherapy with respect to prolonging life. Assessments of the patients' quality of life and psychological adjustment have not traditionally been included in such studies, but there is an increasing recognition of the need for these, and they have been incorporated in some recently designed trials. It is only with this information that a comprehensive evaluation of treatments can be carried out, and more thought needs now to be given to the kinds of measures that are most appropriate in this setting (Endicott, 1984; Gottschalk, 1984). Questionnaires, inventories, and procedures designed for a psychiatric population may not be sufficiently sensitive to detect degrees of distress that fall outside the psychiatric range but are still undesirable, and many of the indices of disturbed mood conventionally employed, such as disturbances in sleep or eating, can be misleading in the context of physical illness.

An issue raised in the conduct of trials, and one that has recently been much debated both in Europe and the United States, is their ethical implications. In routine practice, there are many surgeons who opt for breast conservation, while other surgeons are wary of the consequences of such a conservative approach and still prefer to carry out some form of mastectomy. Similarly, there are surgeons who have already been convinced by the results of the early trials of adjuvant systemic therapy so that they never withhold such treatment in patients with involved axillary nodes while, on the other hand, there remain many surgeons who are frightened by the toxicity of such a policy and never routinely advocate such treatment. No one would question the ethical standing of either of these types of practitioner. Yet, should an individual surgeon faced with a patient with early breast cancer decide, on the toss of a coin, whether she should have her breast conserved or removed, or whether or not she should have toxic combination chemotherapy, it is likely that the majority of the lay public would consider this practice highly dubious. The word *treatment* conjures up the image of the omniscient physician offering the best advice and the benefit of all the latest medical technology. Sadly, it would shatter the popular image of the medical profession if the lay public were aware of the extent to which medical treatment is based on ignorance, intuition, or uncorroborated theory. Much "treatment" could easily be looked on as uncontrolled experimentation. Thus, most physicians and lay people who are familiar with the issue are agreed that properly conducted clinical trials, addressing themselves to areas of genuine uncertainty, are necessary, but we now have to consider the more difficult problem of whether the individual patient should or should not be warned that they are about to enter such a study, and what degree of personal choice can be permitted to her.

Right from the start, we need to make a distinction between an approach that is meant to protect the patient and an approach that is meant to protect the physician. Where there is legislation on clinical trials and a requirement for informed consent, then, in order to protect himself from litigation, the physician is forced to seek such consent. This state of affairs exists in the United States, where patients have to read and sign a very detailed account of what is on offer, together with all the likely and unlikely side effects. Such formulae can be looked on as mechanisms to protect the physician. What should really concern us is how to protect the patient. One risk is that of exposing her to unwarranted and dangerous experimentation. There are, in fact, guidelines and active ethical committees to protect the patient from this, although whether these are sufficiently effective has been argued in a series of articles published in the *Lancet* and *New England Journal of Medicine* (Brewin, 1982; Elkeres, 1982; Schafer, 1982). More controversial is the problem of informed consent, and there are arguments for and against this. These can be summarized as follows. The most popular argument in favor of fully informed consent is respect for another person's right to self-determination. It could also be argued that this approach would improve the patient's knowledge and understanding of the illness and treatment. Full informed consent would also involve the patient in the decision-making process, and this could help ensure cooperation throughout the period of the trial. Finally, in those countries where it is relevant, protection from litigation cannot be dismissed as irrelevant to the patient's well-being, as the physician's own peace of mind may be important for him to practice effectively. The major argument against informed consent is the difficulty that any lay person must face in fully comprehending the disease and in truly understanding the need and mechanism of randomization. Second, full informed consent is likely to undermine the patient's confidence in the physician and cause undue distress and anxiety by admitting that there is uncertainty in the treatment of a potentially fatal disease. Finally, informed consent is likely to interfere with the normal physician-patient relationship, where the patient sees herself as a client seeking the best advice from a professional.

Unfortunately, there is a complete absence of empirical data to help in this debate, as all papers on this topic reflect subjective attitudes to a moral dilemma as argued by physicians, lawyers, and ethicists. The information essential for us to make an educated judgment on these issues concerns the patient's attitudes to informed consent, and this information we do not have. For example, what percentage of patients would accept or refuse entry to a randomized controlled trial with or without full informed consent? What effect would informed consent have on the patient's confidence in their physician and in the physician-patient relationship? Would the expressed uncertainty concerning the best treatment cause additional anxiety and depression, which might itself impair recovery, or would a frank and open discussion between physician and patient cement a relationship based on trust? A clinical experiment to provide such data has recently been launched by the Ludwig Institute for Cancer Research in Sydney, Australia (Tattersall, 1981). Patients with cancer eligible for any one of a number of clinical trials are prerandomized to either a "standard practice" group, who would be handled in a very similar way to the majority of patients entering clinical trials in the United Kingdom, or to a group identified as "total disclosure" who receive full verbal and written information about their disease and the clinical trial that they might enter. The first group are randomized into the clinical trial without foreknowledge. The second group only enter the randomized trial if informed consent is obtained, and, if the consent is refused, the patient is managed as requested. This eventually leads to three groups of patients. One group within a randomized trial without informed consent, another group in the same trial but with informed consent, and a third group having refused consent being managed as they themselves have determined. The numbers of patients consenting to enter into the trial, attitudes of the patients to the physicians and their treatment, attitudes of the patients to informed consent, and states of anxiety and depression before and after the treatment, are being assessed and quantified.

The relative merits of different treatments are still uncertain and, just as individual surgeons tend to prefer some options to others, so many patients have a preference of their own if the facts are made available to them. They may, in particular, be able to make their own "trade off" between quality and quantity of life (Gillie, 1982; Schafer, 1982; Smith, 1982), and some may choose to incur a hypothetical increased risk of recurrence or decreased survival in order to enhance the former. As a recent working party argued: "Though [the patient] has surrendered her body [to the physician] for treatment, however, she has not surrendered her right as an individual to self determination " (Cancer Research Campaign Working Party in Breast Conservation, 1983, p. 3). It has been suggested that if patients are fully informed and allowed choice in clinical trials, then those who enter the trial having accepted the principle of randomization are not a representative group (Brinkley, 1982). Nevertheless, the kinds of bias that are thereby introduced may not be crucial in assessing the physical outcome of treatments. It should be remembered that the designs of clinical trials are derived from research in very different areas, namely agriculture, and they may not be necessary or appropriate in a clinical context (Little, 1983). These authors can offer no easy solution to the dilemma. The real need for controlled and systematic research must be balanced against the right of the patient to be considered as an individual and to be granted a say in decisions about her treatment unless she wishes otherwise. Finally, the problem of informed consent relates, in principle, not only to the conduct of clinical trials but to the more general issue of the extent to which patients should be consulted about their treatment. Few who receive routine care are even aware that there are alternatives (Schmale, Cherry, Morris,

& Henrichs, 1983), and they are thereby deprived of the opportunity to discuss the merits of these with their physicians and of influencing the decision. Whenever the clinician feels that there are realistic alternatives for treatment, it could be argued that he has a moral obligation to inform patients of these, even though it means admitting that he himself does not know which is the best treatment. This does not imply forcing such discussions and decisions on patients. There will be many who prefer to leave things in the clinician's hands, and their needs too can be protected. The working party referred to above suggests the following strategy for obtaining informed consent in clinical trials, but it is one that is more generally applicable: "[A] doctor will carefully prepare the ground for dialogue, but if, at some stage, the patient states explicitly that she does not wish for further information (although she knows that it is available) and tells the physician to proceed as he thinks fit, then his duty to inform further ceases, at least while the patient's attitude remains unchanged" (C.R.C. Working Party, pp. 5-6). Many patients are happy to give their implicit consent to whatever the physician himself thinks is best, but others who would wish to take a more active role and assume some responsibility for their fate should not be denied this opportunity.

Summary

The current model of breast cancer is a deterministic one. Outcomes depend on the micrometastatic spread at the time of treatment, and local treatments are palliative rather than curative. Some clinicians have turned to adjuvant systemic therapy, with the hope of improving survival, but the effectiveness of these treatments has yet to be clearly demonstrated. Recognizing the limitations of the therapies they can offer, clinicians are now becoming increasingly concerned about their costs to the patient in terms of quality of life.

The surgeon who himself has the necessary resources can help the patient to come to terms with her illness and its treatment. But the situation is a complex and difficult one for him also. Some physicians genuinely regard such issues as beyond their province, while some take an impersonal stance toward the patient as a way of managing their own stress. Furthermore, others who would like to take a more personal approach may feel constrained by a lack of the relevant knowledge and skills. Additional support for the breast cancer patient, in the form of the specialist nurse or some alternative intervention, may then be required if the needs of the patient are to be met adequately. When considering the stress of breast cancer, we should not forget the general public, and patients with symptoms whose disease has not yet been diagnosed. Health education should aim to correct overpessimistic misperceptions, and offer appropriate reassurance, and avoid increasing anxiety unnecessarily when advocating behavior change.

Alternative treatments for breast cancer might reduce the morbidity associated with standard procedures, or make the morbidity more acceptable by virtue of their enhanced effectiveness. Clinical trials are necessary to evaluate new treatments, on dimensions of both efficacy and morbidity, but ethical problems are involved in these trials. Should the patient be told that her own treatment is being determined on a random basis, and what degree of choice should she be permitted? On the one hand there is an urgent need for controlled experiments that can offer unambiguous answers to therapeutic dilemmas while, on the other hand, the right of the patient to self-determination, should she so wish, cannot be denied.

References

Abrams, R. O. & Finesinger, J. E. (1953). Guilt reactions in patients with cancer. *Cancer, 6*, 474-482.

Abse, D. W., Wilkins, M. M., Van der Castle, R. L. Dimmock-Buxton, W., Demars, J. P., Brown, R. S. & Kirschner, L. G. (1974). Personality and behaviour characteristics of lung cancer patients. *Psychosomatic Medicine, 18*, 101-113.

Ader, R. (1981). Psychoneuroimmunology. New York: Academic Press.

Aitken-Swan, J. & Easson, E. C. (1959). Reactions of cancer patients on being told their diagnosis. *British Medical Journal*, i, 779-783.

Aitken-Swan, J. & Paterson, R. (1955). The cancer patient: Delay in seeking medical advice. *British Medical Journal*, i, 623-627.

American Cancer Society (1973). Women's attitudes regarding breast cancer. Princeton: The Gallup Organization.

Anderson, E. R. (1973). *The role of the nurse*. Royal College of Nursing, London.

Antonovsky, A. & Anson, O. (1976). Factors related to preventive health behaviour. In J. W. Cullen, B. H. Fox, & R. N. Isom (Eds.), *Cancer The behavioral dimensions* (pp. 35-44). New York: Raven Press.

Apple, D. (1960). How laymen define illness. *Journal of Health and Social Behavior, 1*, 219-225.

Atkins, Sir H., Hayward, J. L., Klugman, D. L., & Wayte, A. B. (1982). Treatment of early breast cancer: A report after ten years of a clinical trial. *British Medical Journal, 2*, 423-429.

Auerbach, S. M. (1973). Trait-state anxiety and adjustment to surgery. *Journal of Consulting and Clinical Psychology, 40*, 264-271.

Averill, J. R. (1973). Personal control over aversive stimuli, and its relationship to stress. *Psychological Bulletin, 80*, 286-303.

Bacon, C. L., Renneker, R., & Cutler, M. (1952). A psychosomatic survey of cancer of the breast. *Psychosomatic Medicine, 14*, 453-460.

Bahnson, C. B. (1969). Psychophysiologic complementarity in malignancies: Past work and future vistas. *Annals of the New York Academy of Science, 164*, 319-333.

Bahnson, C. B. (1980). Stress and cancer: The state of the art. *Psychosomatics, 21*, 975-981.

Bahnson, C. B. & Bahnson, M. B. (1966). Role of the ego defenses: Denial and repression in the etiology of malignant neoplasm. *Annals of the New York Academy of Science, 125*, 827-845.

Bakal, D. A. (1979). *Psychology and medicine: Psychobiological dimensions of health and sickness.* New York: Springer.

Baltrusch, H. J. F. (1963). Problems of research strategy in the psychosomatic approach to malignant disease. In D. M. Kissen & L. L. Le Shan (Eds.), *Psychosomatic aspects of neoplastic disease* (pp. 170-183). Philadelphia: Lippincott.

Bandura, A. (1977). Self-efficacy: Toward a unifying theory of behavioral change. *Psychological Review, 84*, 191-215.

Banks, F. R. & Keller, M. D. (1971). Symptom experience and health action. *Medical Care, 9*, 498-502.

Bard, M. & Sutherland, A. M. (1955). Psychological impact of cancer and its treatment. IV. Adaptation to radical mastectomy. *Cancer, 8*, 656-672.

Baric, L. (1969). Recognition of the "at risk" role: A means to influence health behaviour. *International Journal of Health Education, 12*, 24-34.

Baric, L. (1979). Levels of uncertainty and health actions. In C. R. Bell (Ed.), *Uncertain outcomes* (pp. 173-184). Lancaster: MTP.

Barthrop, R. W., Lazarus, L., Luckhurst, E., Kiluh, L., & Penny, R. (1977). Depressed lymphocyte functioning after bereavement. *Lancet*, i, 384-836

Baum, M. (1982). Will breast self-examination save lives? *British Medical Journal*, i, 142-143.

Baum, M. & Berstock, D. (1982). Breast cancer: Adjuvant therapy. *Clinics in Oncology, 1*, 901-916.

Becker, H. (1979). Psychodynamic aspects of breast cancer: Differences in younger and older patients. *Psychotherapy and Psychosomatics, 32*, 287-296.

Becker, M. H. (1974). The Health Belief Model and sick role behaviour. *Health Education Monographs, 2*, 409-419.

Becker, M. H. & Maiman L. (1975). Sociobehavioral determinants of compliance with health and medical care recommendations. *Medical Care, 13*, 10-24.

Berkowitz, L. & Cottingham, D. R. (1960). The interest value and relevance of fear arousing communications. *Journal of Abnormal and Social Psychology, 60*, 37-43.

Blackwell, B. (1963). The literature of delay in seeking medical care for chronic illnesses. *Health Education Monographs, 16*, 3-32.

Blaxter, M. (1979). Concepts of causality: Lay and medical models. In D. J. Oborne, M. M. Gruneberg & J. R. Eiser (Eds.), *Research in psychology and medicine*: Vol. 2 (pp. 154-161). London: Academic Press.

Bloom, J. R. (1979). Psychosocial measurement and specific hypotheses: A research note. *Journal of Consulting and Clinical Psychology, 47*, 637-639.

Bloom, J. R. (1982a). Social support systems and cancer. In J. Cohen, J. W. Cullen & I. C. Martin (Eds.), *Psychosocial aspects of cancer* (pp. 129-149). New York: Raven Press.

Bloom, J. R. (1982b). Social support, accommodation to stress, and adjustment to breast cancer. *Social Science and Medicine, 16*, 1329-1338.

Blum, L. H. (1977). Health information via mass media: Study of the individual's concepts of the body and its parts. *Psychological Reports, 40*, 991-999.

Blumberg, E. M., West, P. M., & Ellis, F. W. (1954). A possible relationship between psychological factors and human cancer. *Psychosomatic Medicine, 16*, 277-286.

Booth, G. (1964). Cancer and humanism. In D. M. Kissen & L. L. Le Shan (Eds.), *Psychosomatic aspects of neoplastic disease* (pp. 159-169). London: Pitman.

Boreham, J. (1978). The information process in private medical consultations: A preliminary investigation. *Social Science and Medicine, 12*, 409-416.

Boyle, C. M. (1970). Differences between doctors' and patients' interpretations of some common medical terms. *British Medical Journal, ii*, 286-289.

Bransfield, D. D. (1982). Breast cancer and sexual functioning: A review of the literature and implications for future research. *International Journal of Psychiatry and Medicine, 12*, 197-211.

Brewin, T. B. (1982). Consent to randomised treatment. *Lancet, ii*, 919-921.

Briggs, J. E. & Wakefield, J. (1966). Public opinion on cancer: A survey of knowledge and attitudes among women in Lancaster. Manchester: Manchester Regional Committee on Cancer.

Brinkley, D. (1982). A doctor's dilemma. *Experientia, 41* (Suppl.), 267-271.

Brinkley, D. & Haybittle, J. L. (1975). The curability of breast cancer. *Lancet, ii*, 95.

Brown, E. L. (1965). Newer dimensions of patient care. New York: Russell Sage Foundation.

Brown, G. W. (1974). Meaning, measurement, and stress of life events. In B. S. Dohrenwend & B. P. Dohrenwend (Eds.), *Stressful life events: Their nature and effects* (pp. 217-244). New York: Wiley.

Brown, G. W. & Harris, T. (1978). The social origins of depression. London: Tavistock.

Bruhn, J. G. & Trevino, F. M. (1979). A method for determining patients' perceptions of their health needs. *Journal of Family Practice, 8*, 809-818.

Buls, J. G., Jones, I. H., Bennett, R. C. & Chan, D. P. S. (1976). Women's attitudes to mastectomy for breast cancer. *Medical Journal of Australia, 2*, 236-338.

Burish, T. & Lyle, J. (1981). Effectiveness of relaxation training in reducing adverse reactions to cancer chemotherapy. *Journal of Behavioral Medicine, 4*, 65-78.

Byrne, D. (1964). Repression sensitisation as a dimension of personality. In B. A. Maher (Ed.), *Progress in experimental personality research*, Vol. 1 (pp. 169-220). New York: Academic Press.

Byrne, D. G. (1978). Personality, stress, and coronary heart disease. *Medical Journal of Australia, 2*, 469-470.

Byrne, P. S. & Heath, C. C. (1980). Practitioners' use of nonverbal behaviour in real consultations. *Journal of the Royal College of General Practitioners, 30*, 327-331.

Calnan, M. (1984a). The Health Belief Model and participation in programmes for the early detection of breast cancer. *Social Science and Medicine, 19*, 823-830.

Calnan, M. (1984b). Women and medicalisation: An empirical examination of the extent of women's dependence on medical technology in the early detection of breast cancer. *Social Science and Medicine, 18*, 561-569.

Calnan, M. N., Chamberlain, J. & Moss, S. (1983). Compliance with a class teaching B.S.E. *Journal of Epidemiology and Community Health, 37*, 264-270.

Cameron, A. & Hinton, J. (1968). Delay in seeking treatment for mammary tumours. *Cancer, 21*, 1121-1126.

Cancer Research Campaign Working Party in Breast Conservation (1983). Informed consent: Ethical, legal, and medical implications for doctors and patients who participate in randomized clinical trials. *British Medical Journal, i*, 1117-1121.

Cannon, W. B. (1936). The role of emotion in disease. *Annals of Internal Medicine, 9*, 1453-1456.

Caplan, G. (1974). *Support systems and community mental health*. New York: Behavior Publishers.

Caplan, G. (1981). Mastery of stress: Psychosocial aspects. *American Journal of Psychiatry, 138*, 413-420.

Carnevali, D. L. (1966). Preoperative anxiety. *American Journal of Nursing, 66*, 1536-1539.

Cartwright, A. (1964). *Human relations and hospital care*. London: Routledge and Kegan Paul.

Cartwright, A. (1967). *Patients and their doctors*. London: Routledge and Kegan Paul.

Cassel, J. (1974). Psychosocial processes and stress: Theoretical formulation. *International Journal of Health Sciences, 4*, 471-482.

Cassileth, B. R. & Egan, T. A. (1969). Modification of medical students' perceptions of the cancer experience. *Journal of Medical Education, 10*, 797-802.

Cheeseman, E., Baum, M., & Ray, C. (1979). A controlled trial of preoperative counselling for women undergoing breast surgery. *Clinical Oncology, 5*, 194-195.

Chesser, E. S. & Anderson, J. L. (1975). Treatment of cancer: Doctor-patient communications and psychological implications. *Proceedings of the Royal Society of Medicine, 68*, 793-795.

Cline, R. (1983). Interpersonal communication skills for enhancing physician-patient relationships. *Maryland State Medical Journal, 32*, 272-278.

Cobb, B., Clark, R. L., McGuire, C., & Howe, C. D. (1954). Patient-responsible delay of treatment in cancer. *Cancer, 7*, 920-926.

Cobb, S. C. (1976). Social support as a moderator of life stress. *Psychosomatic Medicine, 38*, 300-314.

Cobliner, G. (1977). Psychosocial factors in gynaecological or breast malignancies. *Hospital Physician, 10*, 38-40.

Coppen, A. & Metcalf, M. (1963). Cancer and extraversion. *British Medical Journal, ii*, 18-19.

C.R.C. Working Party (1982). Announcement of breast conservation trial. *Lancet, ii*, 888.

Crisp, A. H. (1970). Some psychosomatic aspects of neoplasia. *British Journal of Medical Psychology, 43*, 313-333.

Darbonne, A. (1967). Crisis: A review of theory, practice and research. *Psychotherapy, 4*, 371-379.

Dattore, P. J., Shontz, F. C., & Coyne, L. (1980). Premorbid personality differentiation of cancer and noncancer groups: A test of the hypothesis of cancer proneness. *Journal of Consulting and Clinical Psychology, 48*, 388-394.

Davis, A. (1960). Uncertainty in medical prognosis: Clinical and functional. *American Journal of Sociology, 66*, 41-47.

Davis, M. S. (1968). Variations in patients' compliance with doctors' advice: An empirical analysis of patterns of communication. *American Journal of Public Health, 58*, 274-288.

Davison, R. L. (1965). Opinion of nurses on cancer, its treatment and curability. A survey among nurses in public health service. *British Journal of Preventive and Social Medicine, 19*, 24-29.

Dean, A. & Lin, N. (1977). The stress-buffering role of social support. *Journal of Nervous and Mental Diseases, 165*, 303-417.

Denton, S. & Baum, M. (1983). Psycho-social aspects of breast cancer. In P. G. Margolese (Ed.), *Breast cancer* (pp. 173-185). New York: Churchill-Livingstone.

Derogatis, L. R., Abeloff, M. D., & Melisaratos, N. (1979). Psychological coping mechanisms and survival time in metastatic breast cancer. *Journal of the American Medical Association, 242*, 1504-1508.

Deutsch, H. (1942). Some psychoanalytic observations in surgery. *Psychosomatic Medicine, 4*, 105-115.

Devitt, J. E. (1976). Clinical prediction of growth behaviour. In B. A. Stoll (Ed.), *Risk factors in breast cancer* (p. 110). London: Heinemann Medical.

Dimatteo, M. R., Taranta, A., Friedman, H. S., & Prince, L. M. (1980). Predicting patient satisfaction from physicians' nonverbal skills. *Medical Care, 18*, 376-387.

Dohrenwend, B. S. & Dohrenwend, B. P. (1974). *Stressful life events: Their nature and effects*. New York: Wiley.

Downie, P. A. (1976). Post-mastectomy survey. *Nursing Mirror, 142*, 65-66.

Dubos, R. (1961). The mirage of health: Utopia, progress and biological change. New York: Doubleday.

Dunkel-Schetter, C. & Wortman, C. B. (1982). The interpersonal dynamics of cancer: Problems in social relationships and their impact on the patient. In H. S. Friedman & M. R. DiMatteo (Eds.), *Interpersonal issues in health care*. New York: Academic Press.

Eardley, A. (1974). Triggers to action: A study of what makes women seek advice for breast conditions. *International Journal of Health Education, 17*, 256-265.

Eardley, A. & Wakefield, J. (1976). Lay consultation by women with a lump in the breast. *Clinical Oncology, 2*, 33-39.

Eisenberg, H. S. & Goldenberg, I. S. (1966). Measurement of quality of survival of breast cancer patients. In J. L. Hayward & R. D. Bulbrook (Eds.), *Clinical evaluation in breast cancer*. London: Academic Press.

Elkeles, A. (1982). Informed consent in clinical trials. *Lancet,* i, 1189.

Elkind, A. K. (1978). "Can it really be cured?": What people ask nurses about cancer. *International Journal of Health Education, 21*, 16-25.

Ellis, D. A., Hopkins, J. M., Leitch, A. G., & Crofton, Sir J. (1979). "Doctor's orders": Controlled trial of supplementary written information for patients. *British Medical Journal,* i, 456.

Endicott, J. (1984). Measurement of depression in patients with cancer. *Cancer, 53* (Suppl. 10), 2243-2249.

Ervin, C. J. (1973). Psychological adjustment to mastectomy. *Medical Aspects of Human Sexuality, 7*, 42-65.

Feder, S. L. (1966). Psychological considerations in the care of patients with cancer. *Annals of the New York Academy of Science, 125*, 1020-1027.

Feifel, H. (1963). Death. In N. Farberow (Ed.), *Taboo topics* (pp. 8-21). London: Prentice Hall.

Felton, B. J. & Revenson, T. A. (1984). Coping with chronic illness: A study of illness controllability and the influence of coping strategies on psychological adjustment. *Journal of Consulting and Clinical Psychology, 32*, 343-353.

Fink, R., Shapiro, S., & Lewinson, J. (1968). The reluctant participant in a breast screening program. *Public Health Reports, 83*, 479-490.

Fishbein, M. & Ajzen, I. (1980). Understanding attitudes and predicting behaviour. London: Prentice Hall.

Fisher, S. (1967). Motivation for patient delay. *Archives of General Psychiatry, 16*, 676-678.

Fletcher, C. M. (1973). Communication in medicine. London: Nuffield Provincial Hospitals Trust.

Forester, B. M., Kornfield, D. S., & Fleiss, J. (1978). Psychiatric aspects of radiotherapy. *American Journal of Psychiatry, 135*, 960-963.

Foucalt, M. (1973). *The birth of a clinic*. London: Tavistock.

Fox, B. H. (1978). Premorbid psychological factors as related to cancer incidence. *Journal of Behavioral Medicine, 1*, 45-133.

Frankenhauser, M. (1976). The role of peripheral catecholamines in adaptation to under-stimulation and over-stimulation. In G. Serban (Ed.), *Psychopathology of human adaptation* (pp. 173-191). New York: Plenum.

Freidson, E. (1961). *Patients' views of medical practice*. New York: Russell Sage Foundation.

Freidson, E. (1970). *Professional dominance: The social structure of medical care*. New York: Atherton.

Freidson, E. (1970). *The profession of medicine: A study in the sociology of applied knowledge*. New York: Dodd-Mead.

French, J. P. & Raven, B. H. (1959). The basis of social power. In D. Cartwright (Ed.), *Studies in social power* (pp. 150-167). Ann Arbor, Michigan: University of Michigan Press.

Freud, A. (1946). *The ego and the mechanisms of defence*. New York: International Universities Press.

Friedman, H. J. (1970). Physician management of dying patients: An exploration. *Psychiatry in Medicine, 1*, 295-305.

Friedman, M. (1969). *Pathogenesis of coronary heart disease*. New York: McGraw-Hill.

Gardner, K. G. (1979). Supportive nursing: A critical review of the literature. *Journal of Practical Nursing and Mental Health Service, 17*, 10-16.

Gilbertsen, V. A. & Wangensteen, O. H. (1962). Should the doctor tell the patient that the disease is cancer? *CA, 12*, 82-86.

Gillie, O. & Panton, L. (1982). Viewpoints on the ethics of clinical experimentation. *Experientia, 41* (Suppl.), 255-266.

Glass, D. C. (1977). Behaviour patterns, stress and coronary disease. Hillsdale, N.J.: Lawrence Erlbaum.

Goffman, E. (1963). *Stigma*. Englewood Cliffs, N.J.: Prentice-Hall.

Gold, M. A. (1964). Causes of patient delay in disease of the breast. *Cancer, 17*, 564-577.

Goldfarb, C., Driesen, J., & Cole, D. (1967). Psychophysiological aspects of malignancy. *American Journal of Psychiatry, 123*, 1545-1553.

Goldsen, R. K. (1963). Patient delay in seeking cancer diagnosis: Behavioral aspects. *Journal of Chronic Diseases, 16*, 427-436.

Goldstein, M. J. (1973). Individual differences in response to stress. *American Journal of Community Psychology, 1*, 113-137.

Goodwin, L. & Taylor, N. (1977). Doing away with the "doctor-nurse game." *Supervisor Nurse, 8*, 25-26.

Gordon, C. (1966). Role theory and illness. New Haven: College and University Press.

Gordon, W. A., Freidenbergs, I., Diller, L., Hibbard, M., Wolf, C., Levine, L., Lipkins, R., Ezrachi, O., & Lucido, D. (1980). Efficacy of psychosocial intervention with cancer patients. *Journal of Consulting and Clinical Psychology, 48*, 743-759.

Gottschalk, L. A. (1984). Measurement of mood and affect in cancer patients. *Cancer, 53* (Suppl. 10), 2236-2242.

Green, L. W. & Roberts, B. J. (1974). The research literature on why women delay in seeking medical care for breast symptoms. *Health Education Monographs, 2*, 129-177.

Greene, W. A. (1954). Psychological factors and reticulo-endothelial disease: I. Preliminary observations on a group of males with lymphomas and leukaemias. *Psychosomatic Medicine, 16*, 220-230.

Greene, W. A. (1965). Disease response to life stress. *Journal of the American Medical Women's Association, 20*, 133-140.

Greene, W. (1966). The psychosocial setting of the development of leukaemia and lymphoma. *Annals of the New York Academy of Science, 125*, 794-801.

Greene, W. A., Young, L. E., & Swisher, S. N. (1956). Psychological factors and reticuloendothelial disease II. Observations on a group of women with lymphomas and leukaemias. *Psychosomatic Medicine, 18*, 284-303.

Greer, S. (1974). Psychological aspects: Delay in the treatment of breast cancer. *Proceedings of the Royal Society of Medicine, 67*, 470-473.

Greer, S. (1984). The psychological dimension in cancer treatment. *Social Science and Medicine, 18*, 345-349.

Greer, H. S. & Morris, T. (1975). Psychological attributes of women who develop breast cancer: A controlled study. *Journal of Psychosomatic Research, 19*, 147-153.

Greer, S., Morris, T., & Pettingale, K. W. (1979). Psychological response to breast cancer: Effect on outcome. *Lancet, ii*, 785-787.

Grinker, R. R. (1966). Psychosomatic aspects of the cancer problem. *Annals of the New York Academy of Science, 25*, 876-882.

Grossarth-Maticek, R. (1980). Psychosocial predictors of cancer and internal diseases: An overview. *Psychotherapy and Psychosomatics, 33*, 122-128.

Grossarth-Maticek, R., Kanazir, D. T., Vetter, H. & Schmidt, P. (1982). Psychosomatic factors in the process of cancerogenesis. *Psychotherapy and Psychosomatics, 38*, 284-302.

Grossarth-Maticek, R., Kanazir, D. T., Schmidt, P., & Vetter, H. (1983). Psychosomatic factors involved in the process of cancerogenesis. Preliminary results of the Yugoslav prospective study. *Psychotherapy and Psychosomatics, 40*, 191-210.

Gruendemann, B. J. (1965). The impact of surgery on body image. *Nursing Clinics of North America, 10*, 635-643.

Gyllensköld, K. (1982). *Breast cancer: The psychological effects of the disease and its treatment*. London: Tavistock.

Haan, N. (1977). *Coping and defending: Processes of self-environment organization*. New York: Academic Press.

Hackett, T. P., Cassem, N. H., & Raker, J. W. (1973). Patient delay in cancer. *New England Journal of Medicine, 289*, 14-20.

Haefner, D. P., Kegeles, S. S., Kirscht, J., & Rosenstock, I. M. (1967). Preventive actions in dental disease, tuberculosis and cancer. *Public Health Reports, 83*, 451-459.

Hagnell, O. (1966). The premorbid personality of persons who develop cancer in a total population investigated in 1947 and 1957. *Annals of the New York Academy of Science, 125*, 846-855.

Hall, J. A., Roter, D. L., & Rand, C. S. (1981). Communication of affect between patient and physician. *Journal of Health and Social Behavior, 22*, 18-30.

Halstead, D. (1981). A problem shared... *Community Care, June 4*, 18-19.

Hamilton, V. (1979). Personality and stress. In V. Hamilton & D. M. Warburton (Eds.), *Human stress and cognition* (pp. 67-114). Chichester: Wiley.

Hammerschlag, C. A., Fisher, S., De Cosse, J., & Kaplan, E. (1964). Breast symptoms and patient delay: Psychological variables involved. *Cancer, 17*, 1480-1485.

Haney, C. A. (1977). Illness behavior and psychosocial correlates of cancer. *Social Science and Medicine, 11*, 223-228.

Hardesty, A. S., Burdock, E. I., Lenn, E. A., & Trachtman (1973). Profile of psychological distress in physical illness. *Proceedings of the Annual Convention, American Psychology Association, 8*, 369-370.

Hardy, R. & Hardy, G. (1979). Patterns of communication to cancer patients: A descriptive analysis. *Journal of the Tennessee State Medical Association, 72*, 656-658.

Henderson, J. G. (1966). Denial and repression as factors in the delay of patients with cancer presenting themselves to the physician. *Annals of the New York Academy of Science, 125*, 856-864.

Henriques, B. (1980). Cancer: A prospective study of patients' opinion and reaction to information about cancer diagnosis. *Acta Chirurgica Scandinavica, 146*, 309-311.

Herzlich, C. (1973). *Health and illness: A social psychological analysis.* London: Academic Press.

Higbee, K. L. (1969). Fifteen years of fear arousal: Research on threat appeals, 1953-1968. *Psychological Bulletin, 72*, 426-449.

Hill, D. J., Todd, P., Ryan, J., Margarey, C. J., Pickford, G., Lickiss, N., Hetzel, B. S., & Krister, S. J. (1975). Retrospective survey of women attending a hospital breast clinic. *Cancer Forum, 6*, 323-328.

Hobbs, P. (1980). Social aspects of breast screening: Indications for health education programmes. *Public education about cancer: Recent research and current programmes* (Vol. 55). Geneva: UICC Technical Report Series.

Hobbs, P., Eardley, A., & Wakefield, J. (1977). Motivation and education in breast cancer screening. *Public Health, 91*, 249-252.

Hobbs, P., Haran, D., Pendleton, L. L., Jones, B. E., & Posner, T. (1984). Public attitudes and cancer education. *International Review of Applied Psychology, 33* (special issue), 565-586.

Hockey, L. (1976). *Women in nursing: A descriptive study.* Edinburgh: Hodder and Stoughton.

Hollender, J., Gonnella, C., & Parker, D. (1979). Functional recovery from cancer surgery: Estimation of expectations. *Archives of Physical and Medical Rehabilitation, 60*, 45-49.

Holmes, T. H. & Rahe, R. H. (1967). The social readjustment rating scale. *Journal of Psychosomatic Research, 11*, 213.

Holroyd, K. A. (1979). Stress, coping and the treatment of stress-related illness. In J. R. McNamara (Ed.), *Behavioral approaches to medicine: Applications and analysis* (pp. 191-226). New York: Plenum Press.

Horn, D. (1956). *Public opinion on cancer and the American Cancer Society: A report of a national sample survey.* New York: American Cancer Society.

Horne, R. L. & Picard, R. S. (1979). Psychosocial risk factors for lung cancer. *Psychosomatic Medicine, 41*, 503-514.

Horowitz, M., Schaeffer, C., Hiroto, D., Wilner, N., & Levin, B. (1977). Life event questionnaires for measuring presumptive stress. *Psychosomatic Medicine, 39*, 413-431.

Horowitz, M. J., Wilner, N., & Alvarez, W. (1980). Signs and symptoms of post-traumatic stress disorder. *Archives of General Psychiatry, 37*, 85-92.

Hovland, C. I., Janis, I. L., & Kelley, H. H. (1953). *Communication and persuasion.* New Haven: Yale University Press.

Huggan, R. G. (1968). Anxiety among women with cancer. *Journal of Psychosomatic Research, 12*, 215-221.

Hughson, A. V. & Cooper, A. F. (1982). Psychological aspects of breast cancer and its treatment. *Practitioner, 226*, 1429-1435.

Hulka, B. S., Knapper, L. L., Cassel, J. C., & Mayo, F. (1975). Doctor-patient communication and outcomes among diabetic patients. *Journal of Community Health, 1*, 15-27.

Idler, E. L. (1979). Definitions of health and illness in medical sociology. *Social Science and Medicine, 13*, 723-731.

Jamison, K. R., Wellisch, D. K., & Pasnau, R. O. (1978). Psychosocial aspects of mastectomy: I. The woman's perspective. *American Journal of Psychiatry, 135*, 432-436.

Janis, I. L. (1958). *Psychological stress*. New York: Wiley.

Janis, I. L. & Feshbach, S. (1953). Effects of fear arousing communications. *Journal of Abnormal and Social Psychology, 48*, 79-92.

Jenkins, C. D. (1966). The semantic differential for health: A technique for measuring beliefs about diseases. *Public Health Reports, 81*, 549-558.

Jenkins, C. D. & Zyzanski, S. J. (1968). Dimensions of belief and feeling concerning three diseases: Poliomyelitis, cancer and mental illness: A factor analytic study. *Behavioral Science, 13*, 372-381.

Johnson, E. M. & Starr, D. E. (1980). A group programme for cancer patients and their family members in an acute care teaching hospital. *Social Work in Health Care, 5*, 335-349.

Johnson, J. E., Fuller, S. S., Endress, M. P., & Rice, V. H. (1978). Altering patients' responses to surgery: An extension and replication. *Research in Nursing and Health. 1*, 111-121.

Johnson, J. H. & Sarason, I. G. (1979). Recent developments in research in life stress. In V. Hamilton & D. M. Warburton (Eds.), *Human stress and cognition* (pp. 205-236). Chichester: Wiley.

Johnson, M. M. & Martin, H. W. (1965). A sociological analysis of the nurse role. In J. K. Skipper & R. C. Leonard (Eds.), *Social interaction and patient care* (pp. 29-39). Philadelphia: Lippincott.

Jones, D. R., Goldblatt, P. O., & Leon, D. A. (1984). Bereavement and cancer: Some data on deaths of spouses from the longitudinal study of Office of Population Censuses and Surveys. *British Medical Journal, ii*, 461-464.

Joyce, C. R. B., Caple, G., Mason, M., Reynolds, E., & Matthews, J. A. (1969). Quantitative study of doctor-patient communication. *Quarterly Journal of Medicine, 38*, 183-194.

Joynt, R. J. (1974). The brain's uneasy peace with tumors. *Annals of the New York Academy of Science, 230*, 342-347.

Kalish, B. J. & Kalish, P. A. (1977). *Journal of Nursing Administration*, 51-57.

Kasl, S. (1974). The health belief model and behavior related to chronic illness. *Health Education Monographs, 2*, 453-454.

Kasl, S. & Cobb, S. (1966). Health behavior, illness behavior, and sick role behavior. *Archives of Environmental Health, 12*, 246-266, 531-541.

Katatsky, M. E. (1977). The Health Belief Model as a conceptual framework for explaining contraceptive compliance. *Health Education Monographs, 5*, 232-242.

Katz, J. L., Weiner, H., Gallagher, T. F., & Hellman, L. (1970). Stress, distress and ego defences. *Archives of General Psychiatry, 23*, 131-142.

Kegeles, S. S., Haefner, D. P., & Kirscht, J. P. (1965). Survey of beliefs about cancer detection and taking papanicolaou tests. *Public Health Reports, 80*, 815-823.

Kellam, S. G. (1974). Stressful life events and illness: A research area in need of conceptual development. In B. S. Dohrenwend & B. P. Dohrenwend (Eds.), *Stressful life events: Their nature and effects*. New York: Wiley.

Kelly, G. A. (1950). *The psychology of personal constructs* (Vols. I & II). New York: Norton.

Kelly, W. O. & Friesen, S. R. (1950). Do cancer patients want to be told? *Surgery, 27*, 822-826.

Kerr, T. A., Schapira, K., & Roth, M. (1969). The relationship between premature death and affective disorder. *British Journal of Psychiatry, 115*, 1277-1282.

Kessel, N. & Shepherd, M. (1965). Health and attitudes of people who seldom consult a doctor. *Medical Care, 3*, 6-10.

Kiecolt-Glaser, J. K., Garner, W., Speicher, C., Penn, G., Holliday, J., & Glaser, R. (1984). Psychosocial modifiers of immunocompetence in medical students. *Psychosomatic Medicine, 46,* 7-14.

Kirscht, J. P., Haefner, D. P., & Eveland, J. D. (1975). Public response to various written appeals to participate in health screening. *Public Health Reports, 90,* 539-543.

Kissen, D. M. (1963). Personality characteristics in males conducive to lung cancer. *British Journal of Medical Psychology, 36,* 27-36.

Kissen, D. M. (1967). Psychosocial factors, personality and lung cancer in men aged 55-64. *British Journal of Medical Psychology, 40,* 29-43.

Kissen, D., Brown, R. F., & Kissen, M. (1969). A further report on personality and psychosocial factors in lung cancer. *Annals of the New York Academy of Science, 164,* 535-544.

Kleiman, M. A., Mantell, J. E., & Alexander, E. S. (1977). R_x for social death: The cancer patient as counsellor. *Community Mental Health Journal, 13,* 115-124.

Klein, R. (1971). A crisis to grow on. *Cancer, 28,* 1660-1665.

Knopf, A. (1974). *Cancer: Changes in opinion after 7 years of public education in Lancaster.* Manchester: Manchester Regional Committee on Cancer.

Knopf, A. (1976). Changes in women's opinions about cancer. *Social Science and Medicine, 10,* 191-195.

Kobasa, S. C. (1982). The hardy personality: Toward a social psychology of stress and health. In G. S. Sanders & J. Suls (Eds.), *Social psychology of health and illness* (pp. 3-32). Hillsdale, N.J.: Lawrence Erlbaum.

Koocher, G. P. (1969). Adjustment and coping strategies among the caretakers of cancer patients. *Social Work in Health Care, 5,* 145-150.

Korsch, B., Freeman, B., & Negrete, V. (1971). Practical implications of doctor-patient interactions: Analysis for paediatric practice. *American Journal of Diseases of Children, 121,* 110-114.

Korsch, B. M. & Negrete, V. F. (1972). Doctor-patient communication. *Scientific American, 227,* 66-74.

Kowal, S. J. (1955). Emotions as a cause of cancer. *Psychoanalytic Review, 42,* 217-227.

Krasnoff, A. (1959). Psychological variables and human cancer: A cross-validation study. *Psychosomatic Medicine, 21,* 291-295.

Kushner, R. (1982). A patient looks at breast cancer at the beginning of a New Decade. In W. McGuire (Ed.), *Breast cancer* (Vol. 4, pp. 95-149). New York: Plenum.

Kutner, B. & Gordan, G. (1961). Seeking care for cancer. *Journal of Health and Human Behavior, 2,* 171-178.

Kutner, B., Makover, H., & Oppenheim, A. (1958). Delay in the diagnosis and treatment of cancer: A critical analysis of the literature. *Journal of Chronic Diseases, 7,* 95-120.

Lacey, J. I. (1967). Somatic response patterning and stress: Some revisions of activation theory. In M. H. Appley & R. Trumbull (Eds.), *Psychological stress: Issues in research* (pp. 14-42). New York: Appleton Century Crofts.

Lancet Editorial (1980). In cancer, honesty is here to stay. *Lancet,* ii, 245.

Langer, E. L., Janis, I. L., & Wolfer, J. A. (1975). Reduction of psychological stress in surgical patients. *Journal of Experimental Social Psychology, 11,* 155-165.

Larsen, K. M. & Smith, C. K. (1981). Assessment of nonverbal communication in the patient-physical interview. *Journal of Family Practice, 12,* 481-488.

Laudenslager, M. L., Ryan, S. M., Drugan, R. C., Hyson, R. L., & Maier, S. F. (1983). Coping and immunosuppression. Inescapable but not escapable shock suppresses lymphocyte proliferation. *Science, 221,* 568-570.

Lauer, P., Murphy, S. P., & Powers, M. J. (1982). Learning needs of cancer patients: A comparison of nurse and patient perceptions. *Nursing Research, 31*, 11-16.

Lawrence, S. A. & Lawrence, A. M. (1979). A model of adaptation to the stress of chronic illness. *Nursing Forum, 18*, 33-42.

Lawson, R. J. (1980). Patients' attitudes to doctors. *Journal of the Royal College of General Practitioners, 30*, 137-138.

Laxenaire, M., Bentz, L. & Chardot, N. (1972). Abord psychologique du malade cancéreux. *Psychotherapy and Psychosomatics, 21*, 306-310.

Lazarus, R. S. (1966). *Psychological stress and the coping process.* New York: McGraw-Hill.

Lazarus, R. S. & Folkman, S. (1984). Coping and adaptation. In W. D. Gentry (Ed.), *The handbook of behavioral medicine* (pp. 282-325). New York: Guildford.

Lazarus, R. S. & Launier, R. (1978). Stress-related transactions between person and environment. In L. A. Pervin & M. Lewis (Eds.), *Perspectives in interactional psychology.* New York: Plenum.

Leavitt, F. (1979). The Health Belief Model and utilization of ambulatory care services. *Social Science and Medicine, 13A*, 105-112.

Lee, E. C. G. & Maguire, G. P. (1975). Emotional distress in patients attending a breast clinic. *British Journal of Surgery, 62*, 162.

Lerner, M. J. (1970). The desire for justice and the reaction to victims. In J. Macauley & L. Berkowitz (Eds.), *Altruism and helping behavior.* New York: Academic Press.

Le Shan, L. (1960). Some methodological problems in the study of the psychosomatic aspects of cancer. *Journal of General Psychology, 63*, 309-317.

Le Shan, L. (1966). An emotional life-history pattern associated with neoplastic disease. *Annals of the New York Academy of Science, 125*, 780-793.

Le Shan, L. & Worthington, R. E. (1956). Some recurrent life-history patterns observed in patients with malignant disease. *Journal of Nervous and Mental Diseases, 124*, 460-465.

Letang, B. W. (1977). Co-ordinated supportive services benefit the breast cancer patient. *Delaware State Medical Journal, 11*, 623-624.

Leventhal, H. (1970). Findings and theory in the study of fear communications. In L. Berkowitz (Ed.), *Advances in experimental social psychology* (Vol. 5). New York: Academic Press.

Leventhal, H., Meyer, D., & Nerenz, D. (1980). The common sense representation of illness danger. In S. Rachman (Ed.), *Contributions to medical psychology* (Vol. 2, pp. 7-30). Oxford: Pergamon Press.

Leventhal, H., Singer, R. P., & Jones, S. (1965). Effects of fear and specificity of recommendations upon attitudes and behavior. *Journal of Personality and Social Psychology, 2*, 20-29.

Leventhal, H. & Watts, J. C. (1966). Sources of resistance to fear—arousing communications on smoking and lung cancer. *Journal of Personality, 34*, 155-175.

Levine, C. N. (1962). Anxiety about illness: Psychological and social bases. *Journal of Health and Human Behavior, 3*, 30-34.

Lewis, F. M. & Bloom, J. R. (1978). Psychosocial adjustment to breast cancer. *International Journal of Psychiatry and Medicine, 9*, 1-17.

Ley, P. (1972). Complaints made by hospital staff and patients: A review of the literature. *Bulletin of British Psychological Society, 25*, 115-120.

Ley, P. (1977). Psychological studies of doctor-patient communication. In S. Rachman (Ed.), *Contributions to medical psychology* (Vol. 1, pp. 9-4). Oxford: Pergamon Press.

Ley, P. (1982). Giving information to patients. In J. R. Eiser (Ed.), *Social psychology and behavioral medicine* (pp. 339-374). Chichester: Wiley.

Ley, P. & Spelman, M. S. (1967). *Communicating with the patient*. London: Staples Press.

Lipowski, Z. J. (1970). Physical illness, the individual and the coping process. *Psychiatry in Medicine, 1*, 91-102.

Little, J. M. (1983). Human experimentation and the physician-patient relationship (editorial). *Surgery, 93*, 600-602.

Lundberg, U., Theorell, T., & Lind, E. (1975). Life changes and myocardial infarction: Individual differences in life change rating. *Journal of Psychosomatic Research, 19*, 27-32.

Macleod-Clark, J. (1981). Communications with cancer patients: Communication or evasion? In R. Tiffany (Ed.), *Cancer nursing update*. London: Balliere Tindell.

Magnusson, D. & Endler, N. S. (1977). Personality at the crossroads. Hillsdale, N.J.: Lawrence Erlbaum.

Maguire, G. P. (1976). The psychological and social sequelae of mastectomy. In J. G. Howells (Ed.), *Modern perspectives in the psychiatric aspects of surgery* (pp. 390-421). New York: Brunner/Mazel.

Maguire, G. P., Lee, E. G., Bevington, D. J., Küchemann, C. S., Crabtree, R. J., & Cornell, C. E. (1978). Psychiatric problems in the first year after mastectomy. *British Medical Journal, i*, 963-965.

Maguire, G. P. & Rutter, D. R. (1976). Training medical students to communicate. In A. E. Bennett (Ed.), *Communication between doctors and patients* (pp. 45-74). London: Oxford University Press.

Maguire, G. P., Tait, A., Brooke, M., & Thomas, C. (1980). Psychiatric morbidity and physical toxicity associated with adjuvant chemotherapy after mastectomy. *British Medical Journal, ii*, 1179-1180.

Maguire, P., Tait, A., Brooke, M., Thomas, C., & Sellwood, R. (1980). Effect of counselling on the psychiatric morbidity associated with mastectomy. *British Medical Journal, ii*, 1454-1456.

Maguire, P., Brooke, M., Tait, A., Thomas, C., & Sellwood, R. (1983). The effect of counselling on physical disability and social recovery after mastectomy. *Clinical Oncology, 9*, 319-324.

Margarey, C. J., Todd, P. B., & Blizard, P. J. (1977). Psychosocial factors influencing delay and breast self-examination in women with symptoms of breast cancer. *Social Science and Medicine, 11*, 229-232.

Margolis, G. J., Carabell, S. C., & Goodman, R. C. (1983). Psychological aspects of primary radiation therapy for breast carcinoma. *American Journal of Clinical Oncology, 6*, 533-538.

Maslach, C. & Jackson, S. E. (1982). Burnout in health professions: A social psychological analysis. In G. S. Sanders & J. Suls (Eds.), *Social psychology of health and illness* (pp. 227-254). Hillsdale, N.J.: Lawrence Erlbaum.

Mason, J. W. (1975). A historical review of the stress field. *Journal of Human Stress, 1*, 6-12.

Mastrovito, R. C. (1974). Cancer: Awareness and denial. *Clinical Bulletin, 4*, 142-146.

McGrath, J. E. (1970). A conceptual formulation for research on stress. In J. E. McGrath (Ed.), *Social psychological factors in stress* (pp. 10-21). New York: Holt, Rinehart & Winston.

McIntosh, J. (1976). Patients' awareness and desire for information about diagnosed but undisclosed malignant disease. *Lancet, ii*, 300-303.

McIntosh, J. (1977). *Communication and awareness in a cancer ward*. London: Croom Helm.

McKeown, T. (1976). The role of medicine: Dream, mirage or nemesis. London: The Nuffield Hospital Trust.

Mead, M. (1949). *Male and female: A study of the sexes in a changing world*. New York: Morrow.

Mechanic, D. (1974). Discussion of research programs on relations between stressful life events and episodes of physical stress. In B. S. Dohrenwend & B. P. Dohrenwend (Eds.), *Stressful life events: Their nature and effects* (pp. 87-98). New York: Wiley.

Mechanic, D. & Volkhart, E. H. (1960). Illness behavior and medical diagnosis. *Journal of Health and Human Behavior, 1*, 86-94.

Meichenbaum, D. & Jeremko, M. E. (1982). *Stress reduction and prevention*. New York: Plenum Press.

Messerli, M. L., Garamendi, C., & Romano, J. (1980). Breast cancer: Information as a technique of crisis intervention. *American Journal of Orthopsychiatry, 50*, 728-731.

Meyerowitz, B. (1980). Psychological correlates of breast cancer and its treatment. *Psychological Bulletin, 87*, 108-131.

Mischel, W. (1968). *Personality and assessment*. New York: Wiley.

Molter, N. C. (1979). Needs of critically ill patients: A descriptive study. *Heart & Lung, 8*, 332-339.

Mood, D. W. & Lick, C. F. (1979). Attitudes of nursing personnel toward death and dying. *Research in Nursing and Health, 2*, 95-99.

Morris, T. (1979). Psychological adjustment to mastectomy. *Cancer Treatment Reviews, 6*, 41-61.

Morris, T., Greer, H. S., & White, P. (1977). Psychological and social adjustment to mastectomy. *Cancer, 40*, 2381-2387.

Morrow, G. R. (1981). *Behavioral treatment of anticipatory nausea and vomiting during chemotherapy*. Washington, D.C.: Annual Meeting American Society for Clinical Oncology.

Morrow, G. R., Craytor, J. K., Brown, J., & Fass, M. (1976). Nurses' perceptions of themselves, cancer nurses, typical, ideal and cancer patients. *Perceptual and Motor Skills, 46*, 1083-1091.

Muslin, H. L., Gyarfas, K., & Pieper, W. J. (1966). Separation experience and cancer of the breast. *Annals of the New York Academy of Science, 125*, 802-806.

Nathanson, C. A. (1977). Sex roles as variables in preventive health behaviour. *Journal of Community Health, 8*, 142-155.

Nerenz, D. R., Leventhal, H., Love, R. R., & Ringler, K. E. (1984). Psychological aspects of cancer chemotherapy. *International Review of Applied Psychology, 33* (special issue), 521-529.

Novack, D. H., Plummer, R., Smith, R. L., Ochitil, H., Morrow, G. R., & Bennett, J. M. (1979). Changes in physicians' attitudes towards telling the cancer patient. *Journal of the American Medical Association, 241*, 897-900.

Obrist, P. (1976). The cardiovascular-behavioral interaction. *Psychophysiology, 13*, 97-107.

Oken, D. (1961). What to tell cancer patients: A study of medical attitudes. *Journal of the American Medical Association, 175*, 1120-1128.

Osborne, S. (1978). The role of the specialist in the breast clinic. *Nursing Times, 74*, 1201-1202.

Pack, G. T. & Gallo, J. S. (1938). The culpability for delay in the treatment of cancer. *American Journal of Cancer, 23*, 443-462.

Palmer, B. V., Walsh, G. A., McKinna, J. A., & Greening, W. P. (1980). Adjuvant chemotherapy for breast cancer: Side effects and quality of life. *British Medical Journal, ii,* 1594-1597.

Parsons, J. A., Webster, J. H., & Dowd, J. H. (1961). Evaluation of the placebo effect in the treatment of radiation sickness. *Acta Radiologica, 36,* 129-140.

Parsons, T. (1951). Illness and the role of the physician. *American Journal of Orthopsychiatry, 21,* 452-460.

Paterson, R. (1955). Why do cancer patients delay? *Canadian Medical Association, 73,* 931-939.

Paterson, R. & Aitken-Swan, J. (1954). Public opinion on cancer: A survey of women in the Manchester area. *Lancet, ii,* 857-861.

Paterson, R. & Aitken-Swan, J. (1958). Assessment of the results of 5 years of cancer education. *Lancet, ii,* 702-712.

Pearlin, L. I. & Schooler, C. (1978). The structure of coping. *Journal of Health and Social Behavior, 19,* 2-21.

Pearson, J. & Dudley, H. A. F. (1982). Bodily perceptions in surgical patients. *British Medical Journal, i,* 1545-1546.

Peck, A. (1972). Emotional reactions to having cancer. *Cancer, 22,* 284-291.

Pender, N. J. (1974). Patient identification of health information received during hospitalisation. *Nursing Research, 23,* 262-267.

Pendleton, D. A. & Bochner, S. (1980). The communication of medical information in general practice consultations as a function of patients' social class. *Social Science and Medicine, 14A,* 669-673.

Perrin, G. M. & Pierce, I. R. (1959). Psychosomatic aspects of cancer: A review. *Psychosomatic Medicine, 21,* 397-421.

Perry, C. (1979). Paternalism as a supererogatory act. *Ethics in Science and Medicine, 6,* 155-161.

Pervin, L. A. & Lewis, H. (1978). *Perspectives in interactional psychology.* New York: Plenum.

Pfefferbaum, B., Pasnau, R. O., Jamison, K., & Wellisch, D. K. (1978). A comprehensive program of psychosocial care for mastectomy patients. *International Journal of Psychiatry in Medicine, 8,* 63-71.

Pike, M. C., Henderson, B. E., Krailo, M. D., Duke, A., & Roy, S. (1983). Breast cancer in young women and use of oral contraceptives: Possible modifying effect of formulation and age at use. *Lancet, ii,* 926-930.

Plaja, A. O., Cohen, L. M., & Samora, J. (1968). Communications between physicians and patients in outpatient clinics. *The Milbank Memorial Fund Quarterly, 46,* 161-213.

Polivy, J. (1977). Psychological effects of mastectomy on a woman's feminine self-concept. *Journal of Nervous and Mental Diseases, 164,* 77-87.

Poole, A. D. & Sanson-Fisher, R. W. (1979). Understanding the patient: A neglected aspect of medical education. *Social Science and Medicine, 13A,* 37-43.

Pratt, L., Seligman, A., & Reader, G. (1957). Physicians' views on the level of medical information among patients. *American Journal of Public Health, 47,* 1277-1283.

Prendergrass, E. P. (1965). Host resistance and other intangibles in the treatment of cancer. *Acta Medica Philippina, 1,* 90-95.

Quint, J. C. (1963). The impact of mastectomy. *American Journal of Nursing, 63,* 88-92.

Rabkin, J. G. & Struening, E. L. (1976). Life events, stress and illness. *Science, 194,* 1013-1020.

Rahe, R. H. & Ranson, R. J. (1978). Life change and illness studies: Past history and future directions. *Journal of Human Stress, 4,* 3-15.

Rakos, R. & Schroeder, H. (1976). Fear reduction in help-givers as a function of helping. *Journal of Counseling Psychology, 23*, 428-435.

Ramsay, M. A. E. (1972). A survey of preoperative fear. *Anaesthesia, 27*, 396-402.

Ray, C. (1977). Psychological implications of mastectomy. *British Journal of Social and Clinical Psychology, 16*, 373-377.

Ray, C. (1980). Breast cancer and its treatment: Psychological implications. In S. Rachman (Ed.), *Contributions to Medical Psychology* (Vol. 2, pp. 153-180). Oxford: Pergamon Press.

Ray, C. (1982). The surgical patient: Psychological stress and coping resources. In J. R. Eiser (Ed.), *Social psychology and behavioral medicine* (pp. 483-507). Chichester: Wiley.

Ray, C. & Baum, M. (1979). The relationship between personality and delay in the presentation of breast lumps. *Clinical Oncology, 5*, 194.

Ray, C. & Fisher, J. (1982). Patients' perspectives on breast cancer. Public Education about Cancer UICC Technical Report Series (Vol. 72, (pp. 14-19). Geneva.

Ray, C., Grover, J., & Wisniewski, T. (1984). Nurses' perceptions of early breast cancer and mastectomy, and their psychological implications, and of the role of health professionals in providing support. *International Journal of Nursing Studies, 21*, 101-111.

Ray, C., Lindop, J., & Gibson, S. (1982). The concept of coping. *Psychological Medicine, 12*, 385-395.

Redfield, J. & Stone, A. (1979). Individual viewpoints of stressful life events. *Journal of Consulting and Clinical Psychology, 47*, 147-154.

Renneker, R. & Cutler, M. (1952). Psychological problems of adjustment to cancer of the breast. *Journal of the American Medical Association, 148*, 833-838.

Renshaw, D. C. (1974). Postsurgical emotional reactions. *Journal of the American Osteopathic Association, 73*, 843-848.

Revenson, T. A., Wellman, L. A., & Felton, B. J. (1983). Social supports as stress buffers for adult cancer patients. *Psychosomatic Medicine, 45*, 321-331.

Reynolds, P. M. (1981). Cancer and communication: Information giving in an oncology clinic. *British Medical Journal*, i, 1449-1451.

Reznikoff, M. (1955). Psychological factors in breast cancer. *Journal of Psychosomatic Medicine, 17*, 96-108.

Roberts, C. M. (1977). *Doctor and patient in the teaching hospital*. Lexington, Mass.: Lexington Books.

Roberts, M. M., Furnival, I. G., & Forrest, A. P. M. (1972). The morbidity of mastectomy. *British Journal of Surgery, 59*, 301-302.

Rogers, R. W. (1975). A protection-motivation theory of fear appeals and attitude change. *Journal of Psychology, 91*, 93-114.

Rogers, R. W. & Mewborn, C. R. (1976). Fear appeals and attitude change: Effects of a threat's noxiousness, probability of occurrence and efficacy of coping responses. *Journal of Personality and Social Psychology, 34*, 54-61.

Rosenstock, I. M. (1960). Gaps and potentials in health education research. *Health Education Monographs, 8*, 21-27.

Rosenstock, I. M. (1966). Why people use health services. *Milbank Memorial Fund Quarterly, 44*, 94-124.

Roth, J. A. (1962). The treatment of tuberculosis as a bargaining process. In A. M. Rose (Ed.), *Human behavior and social processes* (pp. 575-588). London: Routledge and Kegan Paul.

Rothenberg, M. B. (1967). Reactions of those who treat children with cancer. *Paediatrics, 40*, 507-519.

Rotkin, I. D., Quenk, N. L., & Couchman, M. (1965). Psychosexual factors and cervical cancer. *Archives of General Psychiatry, 13*, 532-536.

Rotter, J. B. (1966). Generalized expectancies for internal versus external control of reinforcement. *Psychology Monographs, 80*, Whole No. 609.

Ryan, M. (1979). Ethics and the patient with cancer. *British Medical Journal*, ii, 480-481.

Samora, J., Saunders, L., & Larson, R. F. (1961). Medical vocabulary among hospital patients. *Journal of Health and Human Behavior, 2*, 83-92.

Sanger, L. K. & Reznikoff, M. (1981). Comparison of the psychological effects of breast-saving procedures with the modified radical mastectomy. *Cancer, 48*, 2341-2346.

Satariano, W. A. & Echert, D. (1983). Social ties and functional adjustment following mastectomy: Criteria for research. *Progress in Clinical and Biological Research, 20*, 387-394.

Schachter, S. (1959). *The psychology of affiliation*. Stanford, CA: Stanford University Press.

Schafer, A. (1982). The ethics of the randomized clinical trial. *New England Journal of Medicine, 307*, 719-724.

Schain, W. S. (1978). Guidelines for psychological management of breast cancer: A stage related approach. In H. S. Gallager, H. P. Leis, R. K. Snyderman, & J. A. Urban (Eds.), *The breast* (pp. 465-475). St. Louis: Mosby.

Schain, W., Edwards, B. K., Gorrell, C. R., DeMoss, E. V., Lippman, M. E., Gerber, L. H., & Lichter, A. S. (1983). Psychosocial and physical outcomes of primary breast cancer: Mastectomy versus excisional biopsy and radiation. *Breast Cancer Research and Treatment, 3*, 377-382.

Scher, J. J. L., Brick, N. H., Smalley, R. V., & Joseph, R. R. (1977). Group therapy in a breast cancer clinic. *Proceedings of the American Society of Clinical Oncologists, 18*, 282.

Schmale, A. H. (1969). Panel discussion 3. *Annals of the New York Academy of Science, 164*, 629-632.

Schmale, A. H., Cherry, R., Morris, G., & Henrichs, M. (1983). Psychosocial needs of the cancer patient. *Progress in Clinical and Biological Research, 20*, 375-385.

Schmale, A. H. & Iker, H. (1966). The psychological setting of uterine cervical cancer. *Annals of the New York Academy of Science, 125*, 807-813.

Schmale, A. H. & Iker, H. (1971). Hopelessness as a predictor of cervical cancer. *Social Science and Medicine, 5*, 95-100.

Schmale, A. H., Morrow, G., Davis, A., Illies, E., McNally, J., Wright, G., & Craytor, J. K. (1982). Pretreatment behavioral profiles associated with subsequent psychological adjustment in radiation therapy patients: A prospective study. *International Journal of Psychiatry in Medicine, 12*, 187-195.

Schmid, W. L., Kiss, M., & Hibert, L. (1974). The team approach to rehabilitation after mastectomy. *AORN Journal, 19*, 821-836.

Schonfield, J. (1975). Psychological and life experience differences between Israeli women with benign and cancerous breast lesions. *Journal of Psychosomatic Research, 19*, 229-234.

Scott, D. W. (1983). Anxiety, critical thinking and information processing during and after breast biopsy. *Nursing Research, 32*, 24-28.

Scurry, M. T. & Levin, E. M. (1979). Psychological factors related to the incidence of cancer. *International Journal of Psychiatry in Medicine, 9*, 159-177.

Selye, H. (1956). *The stress of life*. New York: McGraw-Hill.

Shands, H. C. (1966). The informational impact of cancer on the structure of the human personality. *Annals of the New York Academy of Science, 125*, 883-889.

Shands, H. C., Miles, H. H. W., & Cobb, S. (1951). The emotional significance of cancer. *American Practitioner, 2*, 261-265.

Shapiro, S., Venet, W., Strax, P., Venet, L., & Roeser, R. (1982). Ten to fourteen-year effect of screening on breast cancer mortality. *JNCI, 69*(2), 349-355.

Shelp, E. E. (1984). Courage: A neglected virtue in the patient-physician relationship. *Social Science and Medicine, 18*, 351-360.

Shonfield, S. B. (1980). On surviving cancer: Psychological considerations. *Comprehensive Psychiatry, 21*, 128-134.

Shukin, S. (1979). Communication (or make that noncommunication) with doctors. *Nursing, 9*, 89-94.

Silberfarb, P. M., Maurer, L. H., & Crovthamel, C. S. (1980). Psychosocial aspects of neoplastic disease: I. Functional status of breast cancer patients during different treatment regimes. *American Journal of Psychiatry, 137*, 597-601.

Simmons, C. C. & Daland, E. M. (1924). Cancer: Delay in surgical treatment. *Boston Medicine and Surgery Journal, 190*, 15-19.

Sklar, L. S. & Anisman, H. (1979). Stress and coping factors influence tumor growth. *Science, 205*, 513-515.

Sklar, L. S., Bruto, V., & Anisman, H. (1981). Adaptation to the tumor-enhancing effects of stress. *Psychosomatic Medicine, 43*, 331-342.

Smith, A. J. (1982). Doubts about research trials. *Experientia, 41* (Suppl.), 267-271.

Smith, F. B. (1979). *The people's health 1830-1910*. London: Croom Helm.

Sobel, H. J. & Worden, J. W. (1979). The MMPI as a predictor of psychosocial adaptation to cancer. *Journal of Consulting and Clinical Psychology, 47*, 716-724.

Sobel, H. J. & Worden, J. W. (1982). *Helping cancer patients cope: A problem solving intervention program for health care professionals*. New York: B.M.A. Audio Cassettes, Division of Guilford Publication Incorporated.

Solomon, G. F., Amkraut, A. A., & Kasper, P. (1974). Immunity, emotions, and stress. *Psychotherapy and Psychosomatics, 23*, 209-217.

Souhami, R. L. (1978). Teaching what to say about cancer. *Lancet*, ii, 935-936.

Spiegel, D. (1979). Psychological support for women with metastatic carcinoma. *Psychosomatics, 20*, 780-789.

Spiegel, D., Bloom, J. R., & Yalom, I. (1981). Group support for patients with metastatic breast cancer. *Archives of General Psychiatry, 38*, 527-533.

Spielberger, C. D., Auerbach, S. M., Wadsworth, A. P., Dunn, T. M., & Taulbee, E. S. (1973). Emotional reactions to surgery. *Journal of Consulting and Clinical Psychology, 40*, 33-38.

Stavraky, K. M., Buck, C. W., Lott, S. S., & Wanklin, J. M. (1968). Psychological factors in the outcome of human cancer. *Journal of Psychosomatic Research, 12*, 251-259.

Stephenson, J. H. & Grace, W. J. (1954). Life stress and cancer of the cervix. *Journal of Psychosomatic Medicine, 16*, 287-294.

Stillman, M. J. (1977). Women's health beliefs about breast cancer and breast self examination. *Nursing Research, 26*, 121-127.

Stimson, G. & Webb, B. (1965). *Going to see the doctor*. London: Routledge and Kegan Paul.

Stockwell, F. (1972). *The unpopular patient*. London: Royal College of Nursing.

Stoll, B. A. (1981). Neuro and psychoendocrine factors in cancer growth. In B. A. Stoll (Ed.), *Hormonal management of endocrine-related cancer* (pp. 205-219). London: Lloyd-Luke.

Strax, P., Venet, L., Shapiro, S., & Gross, S. (1967). Mammography and clinical examination in mass screening for cancer of the breast. *Cancer, 20*, 2184-2189.

Strickland, B. R. (1978). Internal-external expectancies and health-related behaviors. *Journal of Consulting and Clinical Psychology, 6*, 1192-1211.

Sugar, M. & Watkins, C. (1961). Some observations about patients with a breast mass. *Cancer, 14*, 979-988.

Suls, J. (1982). Social support, interpersonal relations, and health: Benefits and liabilities. In G. S. Sanders & J. Suls (Eds.), *Social psychology of health and illness* (pp. 255-278). Hillsdale, N.J.: Lawrence Erlbaum.

Szasz, T. S. & Hollander, M. C. (1956). A contribution to the philosophy of medicine: The basic models of the doctor-patient relationship. *AMA Archives of Internal Medicine, 97*, 585-593.

Tagliacozzo, D. L. & Mauksch, H. O. (1972). The patients' view of the patients' role. In E. G. Jaco (Ed.), *Patients, physicians and illness* (pp. 172-185). New York: Free Press.

Tarlau, M. & Smalheiser, I. (1951). Personality patterns in patients with malignant tumors of the breast and cervix. *Psychosomatic Medicine, 13*, 118-122.

Taylor, S. E., Lichtman, R. R., & Wood, J. V. (1984). Attributions, beliefs about control and adjustment to breast cancer. *Journal of Personality and Social Psychology, 46*, 489-502.

Tenovus Cancer Information Centre (1972). Public opinion on cancer: A survey of knowledge and attitude in S.E. Wales. Cardiff: Tenovus Cancer Information Centre.

Thomas, C. B. & Duszynski, K. R. (1974). Closeness to parents and the family constellation in a prospective study of five disease states: Suicide, mental illness, malignant tumor, hypertension and coronary heart disease. *Johns Hopkins Medical Journal, 134*, 251-270.

Thomas, C. B., Duszynski, K. R., & Shaffer, J. W. (1979). Family attitudes reported in youth as potential predictors of cancer. *Psychosomatic Medicine, 41*, 287-302.

Torrie, A. (1970). Like a bird with broken wings. *World Medicine, April 7*, 36-47.

Tring, F. C. & Hayes-Allen, M. C. (1973). Understanding and misunderstanding of some medical terms. *British Journal of Medical Education, 7*, 53-59.

Twaddle, A. C. (1969). Health decisions and sick role variations: An exploration. *Journal of Health and Social Behavior, 10*, 105-115.

UICC (1982). *Multidisciplinary project on breast cancer*. Geneva: International Union Against Cancer.

UK Trial of Early Detection of Breast Cancer Group (1981). Trial of early detection of breast cancer: Description of method. *British Journal of Cancer, 44*, 618-627.

Vaillant, G. E. (1976). Natural history of male psychological health. V. The relation of choice of ego mechanisms of defense to adult adjustment. *Archives of General Psychiatry, 33*, 535-545.

Van den Heuvel, W. J. A. (1977). Knowledge and attitudes of 344 women concerning breast cancer and breast self-examination. Public education about cancer, 26, 44-54). Geneva: UICC Technical Report Series.

Veronesi, U., Saccozzi, R., Dei Vecchio, M. et al. (1981). Comparing radical mastectomy with quadrantectomy, axillary dissection, and radiotherapy in patients with small cancers of the breast. *New England Journal of Medicine, 305*(1), 6-11.

Verwoerdt, A. (1972). Psychopathological responses to the threat of physical illness. In Z. J. Lipowski (Ed.), *Psychosocial aspects of physical illness: Advances in psychosomatic medicine* (Vol. 8, pp. 119-141). Basel: S. Karger.

Wabrek, A. J. & Wabrek, C. J. (1976). Mastectomy: Sexual implications. *Primary Care, 3*, 803-810.

Wakefield, J. (1966). Public education about cancer in the Manchester area (NACOSS Occasional Papers, No. 4). London: National Council of Social Science.

Wakefield, J. & Davidson, R. L. (1958). An answer to some criticisms of cancer education. A survey among general practitioners. *British Medical Journal*, i, 96-97.

Watson, M., Greer, S., Blake, S., & Shrapnell, K. (1984). Reaction to a diagnosis of breast
cancer: Relationship between denial, delay and rates of psychological morbidity.
Cancer, *53*, 2008-2012.

Waxenberg, S. E. (1966). The importance of the communication of feelings about cancer.
Annals of the New York Academy of Science, *125*, 1000-1005.

Weinstein, S., Sersen, E. A., Fisher, L., & Vetter, R. J. (1964). Preferences for body parts
as a function of sex, age, and socio-economic status. *American Journal of Psychology*,
77, 291-294.

Weisman, A. D. (1972). *On dying and denying*. New York: Behavioral Publications.

Weisman, A. D. (1976). Early diagnosis of vulnerability in cancer patients. *American
Journal of Medicine and Science*, *271*, 187-196.

Weisman, A. D. & Worden, J. W. (1976). The existential plight in cancer: Significance of
the first 100 days. *International Journal of Psychiatry in Medicine*, *7*, 1-15.

Weiss, J. M., Glazer, H. I., & Pohorecky, L. A. (1976). Coping behavior and neurochemical changes: An alternative explanation for the original "learned helplessness"
experiments. In G. Serban (Ed.), *Animal models of human psychiobiology* (pp.
141-173). New York: Plenum.

Weiss, R. S. (1974). The provisions of social relationships. In Z. Rubin (Ed.), *Doing unto
others* (pp. 17-20). Englewood Cliffs, N.J.: Prentice-Hall.

Wellisch, D. K., Jamison, K. R., & Pasnau, R. O. (1978). Psychosocial aspects of mastectomy: II. The man's perspective. *American Journal of Psychiatry*, *135*, 543-546.

Wenderlein, J. M., Prötzel, T., & Lehrl, S. (1979). Who needs more psychosocial oriented
rehabilitation: Women after breast cancer or women after genital cancer? A socio-
psychological study of 308 women (English summary). *Rehabilitation*, *18*, 187-195.

Wheeler, J. I. & Caldwell, B. M. (1955). Psychological evaluation of women with cancer
of the breast and of the cervix. *Journal of Psychosomatic Medicine*, *17*, 256-268.

White, R. W. (1959). Motivation reconsidered: The concept of competence. *Psychological Review*, *66*, 297-333.

Whitlock, F. A. & Siskind, M. (1979). Depression and cancer: A follow-up study. *Psychological and Medicine*, *9*, 747-752.

Wicker, A. W. (1969). Attitudes versus actions. The relationship of verbal and overt
behavioral responses to attitude objects. *Journal of Social Issues*, *25*, 41-78.

Williams, A. F. & Wechsler, H. (1972). Interrelationship of preventive actions in health
and other areas. *Health Service Reports*, *87*, 969-976.

Williams, E. M., Baum, M., & Hughes, L. E. (1976). Delay in presentation of women
with breast disease. *Clinical Oncology*, *2*, 327-331.

Wilson-Barnett, J. (1978). In hospital: Patients' feelings and opinions. *Nursing Times*, *74*,
29-32.

Wilson-Barnett, J. & Carrigy, A. (1978). Factors influencing patients' emotional reactions
to hospitalization. *Journal of Advanced Nursing*, *3*, 221-229.

Winick, L. & Robbins, G. F. (1977). Physical and psychological adjustment after mastectomy. *Cancer*, *39*, 478-496.

Wirsching, M., Stierlin, H., Hoffman, F., Weber, G., & Wirsching, B. (1982). Psychological identification of breast cancer patients before biopsy. *Journal of Psychosomatic
Research*, *26*, 1-10.

Witkin, M. H. (1978). Psychosexual counselling of the mastectomy patient. *Journal of Sex
and Marital Therapy*, *4*, 20-28.

Wolff, H. G. (1953). *Stress and disease*. Springfield, IL: Charles C Thomas.

Woods, N. F. (1975). Influences on sexual adaptation to mastectomy. *Journal of General Nursing, 4*, 33-47.

Worden, J. W. & Weisman, A. D. (1975). Psychosocial components of lagtime in cancer diagnosis. *Journal of Psychosomatic Research, 19*, 69-79.

Worden, J. W. & Weisman, A. D. (1977). The fallacy in postmastectomy depression. *American Journal of Medicine and Science, 273*, 169-175.

Worden, J. W. & Weisman, A. D. (1980). Do cancer patients want counselling? *General Hospital Psychiatry, 2*, 100-103.

Worden, J. W. (1983). Psychosocial screening of cancer patients. *Journal of Psychosocial Oncology, 1*, 1-10.

World Health Organization (1964). *Prevention of cancer* (WHO Series No. 276). World Health.

Wyler, A. R., Masuda, M., & Homes, T. H. (1968). Seriousness of illness rating scale. *Journal of Psychosomatic Research, II*, 363-374.

Zola, I. K. (1973). Pathways to the doctor: From person to patient. *Social Science and Medicine, 7*, 677-689.

Index